YOUTH WITH EATING DISORDERS

When Food Is an Enemy

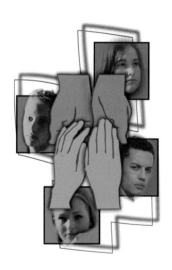

HELPING YOUTH WITH MENTAL, PHYSICAL, AND SOCIAL CHALLENGES

Title List

YOUTH WITH EATING DISORDERS

When Food Is an Enemy

by Noa Flynn

Mason Crest Publishers
Philadelphia

Mason Crest Publishers Inc.
370 Reed Road
Broomall, Pennsylvania 19008
(866) MCP-BOOK (toll free)
www.masoncrest.com

First printing

1 2 3 4 5 6 7 8 9 10

ISBN 978-1-4222-0133-6 (series)

Library of Congress Cataloging-in-Publication Data

Flynn, Noa.
   Youth with eating disorders : when food is an enemy / by
Noa Flynn.
      p. cm. — (Helping youth with mental, physical, and
social challenges)
   Includes bibliographical references and index.
   ISBN 978-1-4222-0144-2
   1. Eating disorders in adolescence—Juvenile literature. I.
Title.
   RJ506.E18F59 2008
   618.92'8526—dc22
2007002669

Interior pages produced by
Harding House Publishing Service, Inc.
www.hardinghousepages.com
Interior design by MK Bassett-Harvey.
Cover design by MK Bassett-Harvey.
Cover Illustration by Keith Rosko.
Printed in the Hashemite Kingdom of Jordan.

Contents

Introduction

We are all people first, before anything else. Our shared humanity is more important than the impressions we give to each other by how we look, how we learn, or how we act. Each of us is worthy simply because we are all part of the human race. Though we are all different in many ways, we can celebrate our differences as well as our similarities.

In this book series, you will read about many young people with various special needs that impact their lives in different ways. The disabilities are not *who* the people are, but the disabilities are an important characteristic of each person. When we recognize that we all have differing needs, we can grow toward greater awareness and tolerance of each other. Just as important, we can learn to accept our differences.

Not all young people with a disability are the same as the persons in the stories. But you will learn from these stories how a special need impacts a young person, as well as his or her family and friends. The story will help you understand differences better and appreciate how differences make us all stronger and better.

—*Cindy Croft, M.A.Ed.*

Did you know that as many as 8 percent of teens experience anxiety or depression, and as many as 70 to 90 percent will use substances such as alcohol or illicit drugs at some time? Other young people are living with life-threatening diseases including HIV infection and cancer, as well as chronic psychiatric conditions such as bipolar disease and schizophrenia. Still other teens have the challenge of being "different" from peers because they are intellectually gifted, are from another culture, or have trouble controlling their behavior or socializing with others. All youth with challenges experience additional stresses compared to their typical peers. The good news is that there are many resources and supports available to help these young people, as well as their friends and families.

The stories contained in each book of this series also contain factual information that will enhance your own understanding of the particular condition being presented. If you or someone you know is struggling with a similar condition or experience, this series can give you important information about where and how you can get help. After reading these stories, we hope that you will be more open to the differences you encounter in your peers and more willing to get to know others who are "different."

—*Carolyn Bridgemohan, M.D.*

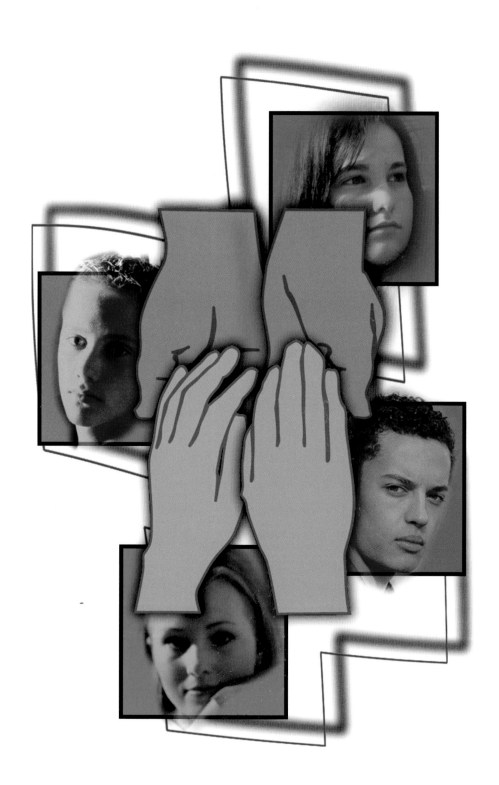

Chapter 1

A New Year, a New Me

Buz-z-z-z!

Oh man, nothing is more annoying than that noise, thought Susan as she reached over to the night table to turn off the alarm. As she lay in bed, she slowly opened her eyes, allowing them to adjust to the sunlight streaming through her bedroom window.

"Susan!" her mother yelled up the stairs. "It's time to get up or you'll be late for your first day."

First day? Susan jumped from the bed. The first day of her junior year of high school. "I'm up. I'm up," she screamed to her mother. Her friends were probably dreading the thought of another year of school, but not Susan. She had a lot—or to be more exact, a lot less—to show her class-mates.

Susan stood before a closet full of new clothes, evidence that she had lost almost forty pounds during the three-month summer vacation. While her friends were off on family vacations, she had gone to "fat camp." They had enjoyed sightseeing and traveling. She had enjoyed—well, "enjoyed" wasn't always exactly the right word—exercising, swimming, biking, hiking, and learning to eat right. While the means of reaching her goal had been hard, she certainly enjoyed the results, a closet of fashionable clothes.

Before going down to breakfast, a meal she had learned at camp was too important to skip, Susan took one more look in the mirror. She had taken extra time on her hair and makeup, and in choosing what to wear. *Today is my chance to wow the other kids.* She was anxious for her friends to see the new Susan.

Whole-wheat toast, fruit, yogurt, and milk were waiting for her on the table. "Thanks, Mom," Susan called to her mother in the kitchen.

"Oh Susan, you look so pretty. That color of blue brings out the blue in your eyes." Susan's mom sat down with her daughter. "Are you excited? A bit nervous?"

Susan hadn't been able to see her friends since she got home from camp. They were all away when she left, and she hadn't gotten home until a couple of nights ago. "I guess I'm more excited than nervous. I just told Gina and Anne that I was going to camp. I didn't tell them what kind of camp."

Gina, Anne, and Susan had been friends since elementary school. They enjoyed doing the same things—shopping, IM-ing each other, going to movies, and eating. At camp, Brenna, one of the camp counselors, had asked the campers to write down the types of things they liked doing with their friends. Susan tried to be honest, so she wrote down "going out for pizza," "eating Chinese," "making cookies"; she had to admit she was surprised about how much of their time she and her friends spent doing food-related things. For some reason, though, Gina and Anne never seemed to gain any weight. No, that was Susan's problem alone. But today, she would show them her new look.

"We're going to the coffee shop after school," Susan called to her mother as she went out of the door.

At camp she had learned how important exercise would be to keeping off the forty pounds she'd left there. So she resolved to walk to school. Usually, her mom dropped her off on her way to work. *No more*, Susan vowed. She had worked hard to get this new body, and she was going to do whatever she needed to keep it.

"Susan?" she heard the familiar voices of Gina and Anne call out to her. "Suz, is that really you?" Gina looked at her as though she had grown another head. "Great outfit, girl! And you look fantastic." Clothes were important to Anne, so Susan wasn't surprised when her outfit got more attention from Anne than her new body. *Sheez! Anne has never commented on my clothes before. I'm liking this attention.* "What happened to you, Susan? You're not sick or anything are you?" asked Gina, whose mother-hen qualities were one of her most endearing features.

"No ladies, I'm not sick. Actually, for the first time in a really long time I am healthy. While you guys were lounging around, I was at a special camp learning to eat better."

"You went to *fat camp!*" laughed Anne. Anne didn't always think before she spoke, and Gina, as usual, smacked her on the arm.

"Anne!" Gina scolded.

"I'm sorry, Susan. That was really rude," Anne quietly apologized.

"It's okay, Annie," Susan said. "That's what it was, after all. And this is the result." Laughing, Susan spun around, showing off her new look. Unfortunately, she spun right into Brooke Ford, *the* Brooke Ford—homecoming queen, prom queen, head cheerleader, and so on, and so on, and so on. Worried about what Brooke might have heard, Susan quickly apologized.

"It's Susan, isn't it? I think we've been in some classes together." Susan was impressed that Brooke knew her name. She was a year ahead of Susan, but they had been in some of the same classes. They certainly weren't friends. After all, they had different friends. Brooke was super-popular, had super-good looks, and was super-wealthy—all things Susan was not. Brooke was staring at her, as though she knew something was different, but she couldn't quite put her finger on what it was. "That's all right," Brooke said slowly, still trying to figure out what was different, "Hey, I'll see you around."

Susan, Gina, and Anne stood there shocked. "She'll see you around?" Gina finally said.

"Wow, I guess your look wasn't the only thing that changed," Anne added.

Susan just smiled. *Maybe everything about my life will change!*

After school the three friends met at the coffee shop, just as they had last year. This time, though, Susan had a plain coffee and no pastry—not the double latte and the pastry of the day that she had ordered almost every day after school last year. Anne and Gina had their usuals, but that didn't bother Susan.

This was the first year in the entire time they had known each other that they didn't have at least one class together, so now they had an entire day to catch up on. "How'd it go, skinny?" Anne asked between slurps of her latte.

"Good, really good," Susan replied with a sigh of contentment. "I was kind of nervous about how people would react, but everyone was really nice. I even got a whistle in the hall—and it was serious." Boys had whistled at Susan before, but it was always mean-spirited, guys making fun of her. This time, though, it was the real thing. Someone thought she was hot.

"Susan, how did you lose all that weight?" Gina asked. "I know you went to camp, but how did that help you? I mean, you really look great, and it's not just the clothes."

Susan sighed. "Well, it didn't happen all at once. Brenna, she was one of the counselors, told us that we didn't gain it all at once so we shouldn't expect to lose it all at once. We learned that some of us have reasons for eating that have nothing to do with being hungry."

"Why eat when you're not hungry?" Anne asked, but Gina sent her *that* glance that told Anne she said something inappropriate. "I'm sorry, Suz," Anne apologized for the second time that day.

"It's all right. That's something many people don't understand. Some people eat because they're bored. Others eat because they're lonely. Stress can also make people eat when they're not really hungry."

"So, why did you eat?" Anne asked.

Gina shook her head. "Sheez, Anne."

Susan giggled. "No, really, it's all right. It helps to talk about it. It reminds me what I learned." Anne glanced at

Gina and gave her a smug smile. Gina just shook her head again. Then they both turned to Susan, waiting for her answer.

"I guess habit was one reason. Whenever we get together, we eat."

Anne and Gina looked at each other, guilt written on their faces. Immediately, Susan realized that they had misunderstood what she was saying. "Guys, it's not your fault. It's no one's fault but mine—but I didn't really know any better. Plus, Brenna thinks that I might have turned to food for comfort when my father and Peter died."

Gina reached over and put her hand on Susan's. Anne put her arm around her friend's shoulders. Susan's father and brother had died a few years ago, her father from cancer and her brother, two months later, in an auto accident. It had been a hard time for Susan and her mother.

"Oh, Susan. I can understand that. They do call it comfort food after all." Anne gave Susan a small smile. This time, Gina did nothing to contradict Anne.

"Anyway," Susan continued, "I gained weight for a lot of different reasons, and I finally decided to do something about it."

"But why now?" Gina asked.

"I don't know. It just seemed to be the time. It was getting harder for me to go up and down stairs. I dreaded PE, especially those gym suits." All three girls nodded in shared disgust at the ugliness of the gym suits. "And, well, to be honest, I was tired of being made fun of. The laughing, the name-calling, the nasty notes about how fat I am—was." Susan paused and took a big breath, "I never told you guys, or anyone else, but I actually thought of killing myself because of the teasing."

Gina and Anne looked at each other. They had had no idea their friend felt so awful. Gina hugged Susan, "I had no clue things were so bad for you. You always seemed so happy, like you had no cares in the world."

Anne reached over and touched Susan on the arm. "Why didn't you say anything, Susan? We're your friends, we would do anything for you."

Embarrassed, Susan looked at the two people she had known for so long. They really did care about her, and now she was afraid she'd sent them both on a major guilt trip. "Now, ladies, that's in the past. This is a new year, and I'm a new person. We're not going to dwell on wouldas, couldas, and shouldas. I've learned how to channel emotions away from destructive eating patterns and how to make better food choices. So, we can still do the same things we've always done—including eating. I'll just choose more healthful foods and drinks." She glanced from her coffee to her friends' lattes. "And I might suggest we go bowling, swimming, or hiking sometimes instead of shopping."

A loud "ugggh," came from Anne's direction.

"Well, maybe just once in a while," Susan laughed.

"Hi, Mom. I'm home." Susan threw her books on the hall table and went into the kitchen. Her mother was leaning into the refrigerator, pulling out a variety of vegetables to prepare for dinner.

"Hi, honey. How was school? Was everyone surprised by the 'new you'?"

"School was fine. Gina and Anne were sure surprised. I had to explain fat camp to them after school." Susan's mother rolled her eyes at the phrase "fat camp." Susan knew her mother hated that term.

"Oh, Susan. You had a call a while ago. I wrote a note and put it . . . now where did I put it? Oh, it's on the bulletin board. Someone named Brooke?"

Brooke? Susan knew only one Brooke—Brooke Ford. But she had no idea why Brooke would be calling her.

While she crunched on carrots and celery, Susan picked up an old issue of *People* from the stack of magazines that had accumulated in a basket on the kitchen floor. She leafed through it idly, pausing to skim an article that claimed Nicole Richie had an eating disorder.

Susan looked at the photographs that accompanied the article. The actress was so skinny that Susan could see the curve of her hipbones jutting out beneath her jeans and there were little shadowy hollows underneath her cheek-bones. Susan touched her own hips with a rueful grin. No one was ever going to accuse her of having anorexia! Even the new and improved Susan still had a fair amount of flesh cushioning her bones.

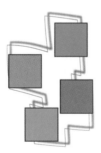

What Is an Eating Disorder?

It is natural to be concerned about your weight. Working to reach and maintain a healthy weight is important for everyone, particularly in a culture where obesity is so prevalent. Being overweight can have dangerous health consequences.

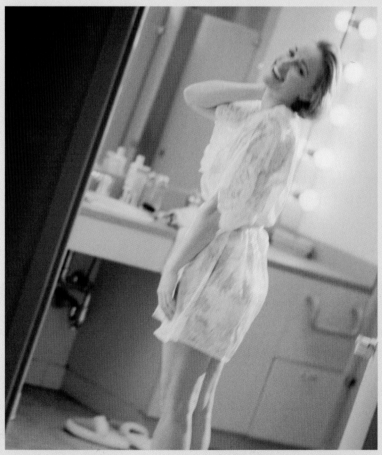

Maintaining a healthy weight is important. Obsessing over every pound is not.

When a healthy concern about your weight crosses the line and becomes an *obsession*, however, it is necessary to seek professional help. But what exactly *is* an eating disorder?

According to the National Institute of Mental Health, eating disorders are psychiatric conditions, "real, treatable medical illnesses in which certain *maladaptive* patterns of eating take on a life of their own." These illnesses may include an unhealthy limitation of food and extreme concern about body shape and weight.

Substance Abuse and Eating Disorders

In 2004, the National Center on Addiction and Substance Abuse issued a report on the similarities between substance abuse and eating disorders. They found the following shared risk factors and characteristics:

Substance Abuse and Eating Disorders	
Shared Risk Factors	**Shared Characteristics**
Occur in times of transition or stress	Obsessive preoccupation, craving, compulsive behavior, secretiveness, rituals
Common brain chemistry	
Common family history	
Low self esteem, depression, anxiety, impulsivity	Experience mood altering effects, social isolation
History of sexual or physical abuse	
Unhealthy parental behaviors and low monitoring of children's activities	Linked to other psychiatric disorders, suicide
Unhealthy peer norms and social pressures	Difficult to treat, life threatening
Susceptibility to messages from advertising and entertainment media	Chronic diseases with high relapse rates
	Require intensive therapy

Source: National Center on Addiction and Substance Abuse, www.casacolumbia.org.

History of Eating Disorders

Although eating disorders might seem to be a recent problem, they have been a recorded part of society since at least the thirteenth century. Between the thirteenth and sixteenth centuries, some people were admired for their apparent ability to survive without food or drink. This condition was called the anorexia miribilis, meaning religious miracle. Fasting—going

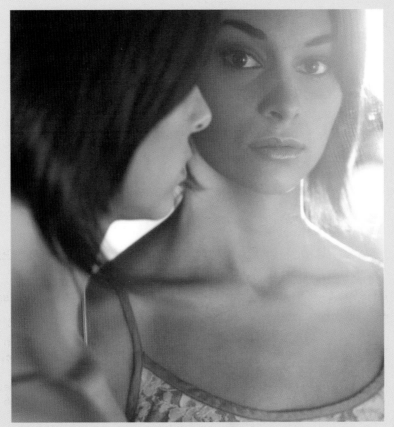

An eating disorder may include unhealthy patterns of eating and an extreme concern about body shape and size.

without food or liquid—was seen as a method of showing one's faith and *subservience* to God.

It was not until the late 1800s that medical professionals began to see this condition as a medical problem rather than a sign of extreme religiosity. In 1873, London physician Sir William Withey Gull gave the condition its name—anorexia nervosa—and established the first *criteria* used to diagnose the disorder.

During the late eighteenth and early nineteenth centuries, being thin became fashionable, and many women went to extremes to be so. Before, being larger was a sign of wealth; plenty of flesh meant the person also had plenty of money for food, while members of the working class were often underfed and *emaciated*. However, as society developed and the cost of producing food decreased, the trend reversed. The upper classes began to believe that "thin was in," so the amount of food eaten—particularly by women—decreased dramatically. (Some women even had ribs removed to achieve that tiny, tiny waistline.) Now, members of the working class weighed more and were looked down on for it.

Today, media emphasis continues to be on a thin, waiflike appearance. Many actresses walking the "red carpet" and models parading down the catwalk appear emaciated; some have even referred to such models as walking skeletons.

While working on *Growing Pains*, actress Tracy Gold developed an eating disorder that caused her to miss many episodes. Sadly, she hasn't been the only one to whom a director or studio executive has

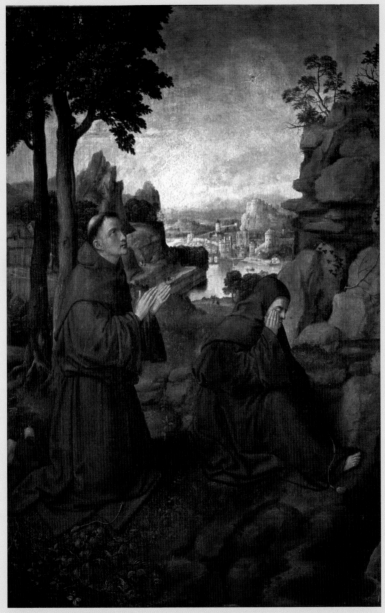

Between the thirteenth and sixteenth centuries, surviving without food and drink was admired as showing one's faith and commitment to God.

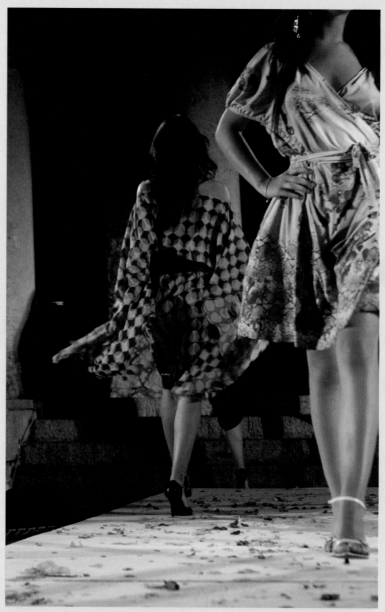

Today, runway models and actresses contribute to the idea that extremely thin equals beautiful.

mentioned that perhaps she needs to lose a few pounds. In many cases, these are teenagers going through a perfectly normal growth spurt. But in much of Hollywood today, there's no excuse for gaining weight.

Famous People Who Have Had an Eating Disorder

Christy Henrich—gymnast (died from complications of her disorder in 1994)

Diana, Princess of Wales

Elton John—musician

Jamie-Lynn Sigler—actress

Jane Fonda—actress, activist, writer, exercise guru

Karen Carpenter—singer (died from complications of her disorder in 1983)

Mary Kate Olsen—actress

Paula Abdul—singer/dancer

Richard Simmons—exercise/diet guru

Tracy Gold—actress

What Is Body Image?

For most of us, when we look in the mirror we pretty much see ourselves how we physically are—warts and all. Perhaps your nose isn't quite as you'd like, or the extra helpings you had at Thanksgiving are showing up around your waist. Still, you have a realistic picture of what your body looks like. According to the Web site womenshealth.gov, body image is:

- How you perceive your physical appearance.
- How you feel about your appearance.

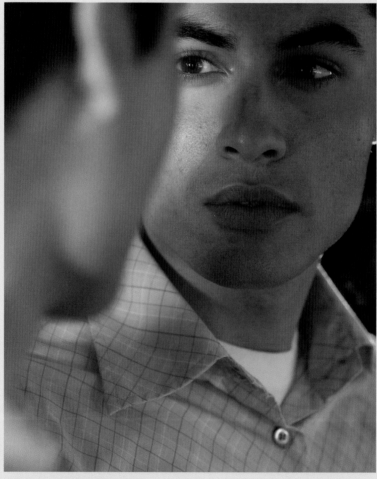

Someone battling an eating disorder may have a distorted view of his own body. He may look in the mirror and see a totally different person than others see.

- How you feel about your body.
- How you think others see you.

For people with anorexia and bulimia, perception of body image is drastically inaccurate. The individual might look in the mirror and "see" a seriously overweight person, when in truth, she is severely undernourished. We've all heard a thin person say, "I'm just so fat." Well, while that is a gross exaggeration (and perhaps said by someone simply looking for reassurance), the person with anorexia or bulimia may truly perceive herself as overweight. Combating an inaccurate body image can be a challenge in the treatment process.

According to the Wellesley College Health Service (cited on www.4womangov/bodyimage/index.cfm):

Our body image is formed out of every experience we have ever had—parents, role models, and peers who give us an idea of what it is like to love and value a body. Image is formed from the positive and the negative feedback from people whose opinions matter to us. It is also the way we ourselves have perceived our body to fit or not fit the cultural image.

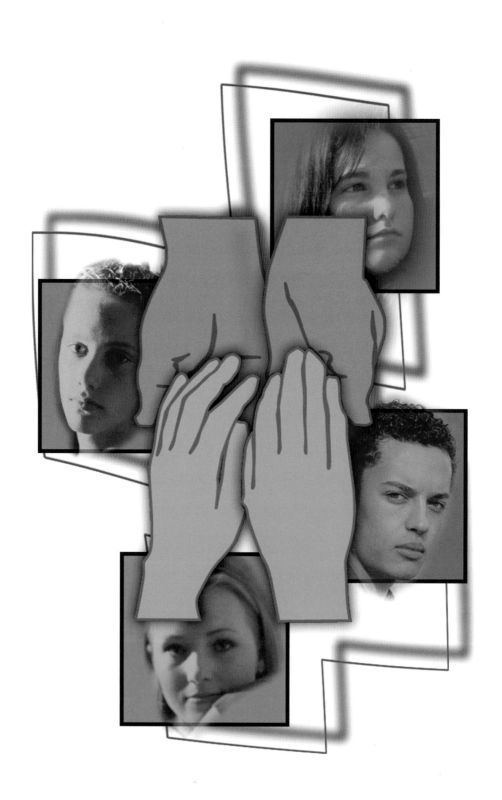

Chapter 2

A New Friend?

Susan paid the cafeteria lady and headed toward her usual lunch table. She had called Brooke last night, but Brooke wasn't home. Susan had to admit that she wasn't surprised. After all, Brooke is one of the most popular kids in school.

"Susan, what are you doing after school?" Gina asked. Gina, Anne, and Susan had been eating lunch together for as long as any of them could remember.

"Oh, I have to go straight home. Mr. Paulson assigned a major research paper."

"When's it due? Let's go to the mall. Do you really have to start the paper already?" Anne asked.

"Well, it's not due for a few weeks, but I want to get a head start on it."

Gina shook her head and started to laugh. "But Suz, you never start your papers and stuff until a day or so before they're due. It's tradition." Anne, and even Susan, had to laugh at that; they all knew that Gina was speaking the truth.

"Oh, come on now," laughed Susan, "that was the *old* Suz. The new and improved me is trying to do better." Anne's eyebrows went up in a "huh," and Gina just looked at her. "Ladies, at fat camp I learned a lot about me and why I overeat."

"Didn't you say it had to do with what happened to your dad and brother?" asked Anne. Gina nodded.

"Well, that is one of the reasons," Susan explained, "but there are many others. One of the reasons people overeat— including me—is stress. So, my goal is to reduce stress, and one of the things that stresses me most is doing my homework at the last minute. I figure if I chop up Paulson's assignment into pieces, I can get the paper done without extra stress." Susan had listened carefully to the suggestions made by Brenna and the other counselors at camp. She hoped this one would work for her.

"Well, it makes sense," agreed Gina, "but does it have to start today?"

Anne's eyes widened and her mouth fell open in surprise at Gina's suggestion. "Gina," she sputtered, "are you trying to sabotage Susan's plan?"

Gina shook her head and opened her mouth to apologize. The three friends looked at each other, and then burst out laughing. For once, Anne had turned the tables on Gina.

After school, Susan went to the library to begin researching her paper. *Maybe I could wait a day or so to start working on this. It'd be fun to go to the mall,* Susan thought as she sat at the library table and looked over the list of suggested topics prepared by her history teacher. None of them looked very exciting; *at least not as exciting as a trip to the mall,* Susan concluded.

"Susan, I thought I saw you come in here." Brooke Ford plopped her books on the library table, loud enough to bring a disapproving scowl from the librarian. Brooke mouthed, "Sorry," in the direction of the librarian and sat down across from Susan. "Sorry I wasn't home when you called," she whispered, "but Scott called, and well, you know how it is."

No, Brooke, I don't know how it is. I don't have a boyfriend, so I don't know how it is, thought Susan. She opted to say out loud, "That's all right, Brooke. Mom said you called; I was just returning your call."

Brooke smiled and leaned forward so she wouldn't have to whisper too loudly. "Susan, you look really great. How did you lose so much weight so quickly?" She looked to make sure no one was listening in, and came even closer to Susan. "What did you use?"

Susan leaned back in her chair, trying to regain some personal space. "Brooke, it wasn't so fast. I started watching what I was eating before school ended last year. Then, I went to a camp that helps teens with food issues. I learned to eat better—especially more healthfully—and the importance of exercise. I didn't *use* anything."

Susan thought Brooke looked as though she had slapped her in the face when she finished her explanation. Brooke rested her chin on her hand. "You mean there wasn't any meds or anything?"

"No, Brooke, just sensible eating and exercise. We learned there are no long-lasting shortcuts. Why are you asking, anyway?"

Brooke looked around, again making sure no prying ears were trying to hear what she and Susan were discussing. "Well, I've put on a few pounds—okay, more than a few."

Susan looked up and down Brooke's slim body. If the prom queen had gained weight, she certainly couldn't see it.

"I need to nip this weight thing in the bud, before it gets out of hand, like it did with you." Brooke's voice trailed off as she realized what she had said. "I'm sorry, Susan. I didn't mean that like it sounded."

"It's all right, Brooke. I'm sure you didn't." Susan even managed a small smile as she half-heartedly tried to reassure Brooke. "No, there wasn't any magic pill or anything. Actually, Brenna—she was one of the counselors—said that most meds only provide a short-term solution. The same with fad diets. But Brooke, you look great—as always."

Brooke sighed. "Thanks, Susan, but I feel fat. I can feel every ounce of those extra pounds. It's even affecting my cheering. I can't jump as high."

Well, at least you can jump, thought Susan. At her heaviest, she had found even walking difficult; she would have never considered jumping. Besides, if she had jumped, Susan was sure that she'd have heard snickers and comments about the Richter Scale.

"But what about all those stars in Hollywood who lose weight really fast?" Brooke persisted. "Or those commercials that advertise pills and stuff that will help you drop pounds fast? Did you try them? Don't they work?"

"Well, Brenna says that some of them do work," Susan answered, "but only for a while. At first, you lose mostly water weight. After that, losing the pounds can be really slow going. Oh, and I'm sure you've heard about low-carb and high-protein diets." Brooke nodded. "You can lose weight on those diets, but they're not really a healthy way to go either."

"What do you mean?" Brooke was clearly skeptical. "Low-carb is all over the place. There are even shelves in the grocery store dedicated to low-carb stuff."

"Sure," Susan replied, "but that doesn't mean they're healthy. Sheez, all the things that help make people fat are all over the place, too. Brenna reminded us that our bodies need all kinds of things in order to be healthy. You know, the stuff we've been taught forever in health classes? Well, if you only eat one thing, or one group of foods, then your body can suffer from lack of nutrients."

"Isn't that where vitamins and other supplements come in? You just take a vitamin pill—and then you don't have to worry about the calories that go along with the food."

"Yeah, but it's always best to get vitamins and stuff naturally, not from pills or liquid supplements. Oh, and once you go off those diets and start eating other foods, well, the weight can come back. Brooke, I learned that diets just don't work over the long term. If someone needs to lose weight, she needs to take a good look at what she eats, come up with a food plan that works for her, and then exercise. Brenna always said that you don't gain the weight in a week, so you can't expect to take it off in a week."

Brooke sighed, and Susan knew that she hadn't told Brooke what she had hoped to hear. "Oh well, just thought I'd ask." Brooke grabbed her books and got up to leave. "I gotta run. I'm supposed to meet the girls at the coffee shop. Hey, you should join us."

Susan gathered up her papers and stood up to go with her new friend. But she wasn't fast enough. "Well, sometime then. See you, Susan," said Brooke as she quickly headed for the library door.

Well, I might as well go home. I don't feel like studying anymore. Susan walked home alone.

"Hey, Suz," called Gina as she and Anne ran to catch up with Susan as she walked to school the next day. "We missed you yesterday."

"Yeah, I probably should have come with you. I didn't exactly get much work done." Susan was sure that Brooke wouldn't appreciate her telling Gina and Anne about their conversation. And she was too embarrassed to tell her friends that she had misunderstood Brooke's "invitation" to join her and her friends.

"Well, can you come to the coffee shop after school this afternoon?" Anne asked. "Or we can do something else if you want. Let's just hang out."

As the girls crossed the parking lot, Scott Lyle's Mustang pulled in and parked. Brooke got out of the passenger side, and gave Susan a quick little smile when they made eye contact. Susan took a good look at the impeccably dressed Brooke. *I'm sorry, Brooke,* thought Susan, *but I sure don't see where you have any problem with weight.*

"So Suz, what do you think?" Gina interrupted Susan's train of thought.

"Sure, let's go to the coffee shop," answered Susan. *Studying can wait another day.*

After school Gina, Anne, and Susan sat in the coffee shop. Again, Susan was having plain coffee and skipped the pastry. Even Gina and Anne decided not to have pastries, but they did have double lattes. "So, Anne and Susan, do you want to go bowling this weekend?" Anne and Susan looked at each other and then at their friend. "Well, you said we might be going bowling sometime, and I thought now would be good," Gina went on, trying to sell her friends on the idea.

"I'm game," replied Anne.

"So am I," echoed Susan, "but I thought I'd have to be the one to bring it up."

"Sheez, Suz, do you think you're the only one who can change?" Gina grinned at Susan.

The girls sat finishing their coffees and making plans for bowling. The door to the coffee shop opened, and in walked Scott, Brooke, Sydney Pope, Jeff Michaels, Jessica Myers, and Paul Breen—the popular clique. Sydney and Jessica were on the cheerleading squad with Brooke. Jeff and Paul were their boyfriends. Jeff was on the football team with Scott; Paul was on the wrestling team. Everyone in the coffee shop turned and looked when the group walked in. After all, they were a hard group to miss, laughing and talking loudly whenever they entered a room.

Susan and Brooke gave each other a little smile of acknowledgment. On the group's way to a table, Brooke quickly dropped a folded piece of paper on the table in front of Susan. She unfolded the note: *Susan, Thanks for the info. I think I've found a solution to my problem. Let's get together some time.* Her signature was written with a flourish that a name like Brooke—and not a name like Susan—evokes.

"What's that all about?" Gina asked, looking over at the "popular" table.

"Oh nothing," answered Susan. "I just helped her with something the other day at the library." *At least I hope I helped her,* Susan mused, *but I'd sure like to know what she means by a "solution."*

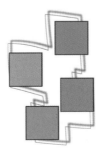

There are three major types of eating disorders: anorexia nervosa, bulimia nervosa, and binge eating.

Anorexia Nervosa

Anorexia nervosa, or anorexia, is deliberate starvation with the purpose of losing weight. Along with lack of food, the person with anorexia can over-exercise and may use laxatives or *diuretics* to speed up weight loss. The individual has a distorted image of his or her body, and the fear of becoming fat controls all the person's actions. Left untreated, anorexia can lead to physical and psychological damage, and even death.

In 2006, the American Psychiatric Association reported that between 0.5 percent and 3.7 percent of females will become anorexic at some time during their lives. Although anorexia can occur at any age, for most, its onset will take place during puberty or young adulthood. Most people with anorexia are female and Caucasian. Those who participate in activities that place importance on being thin—such as gymnastics, modeling, and ballet—also tend to develop anorexia at a higher rate.

To be diagnosed with anorexia, someone must:

• be 15 percent below their ideal weight as indicated by the Metropolitan Life Insurance tables, growth charts, or the Centers for Disease Control and Prevention (CDC) *body mass index* [BMI].

• have an extreme fear of being fat, even when underweight.

- have a distorted body image.
- deny having an eating disorder problem although underweight.
- miss at least three menstrual periods in a row.

They may also **binge** and *purge*.

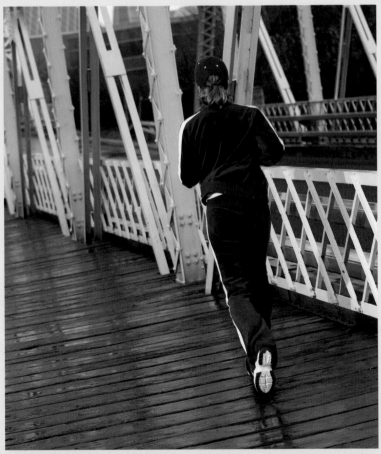

A person with anorexia often over-exercises along with under-eating.

Calculating Body Mass Index

To figure out your body mass index if you are over eighteen, use the following equation:

weight in pounds ÷ [height in inches]^2 x 703.

If your BMI is	you're classified as
<18.5	underweight
18.5–24.9	normal*
25.0–29.9	overweight
30.0 and above	obese

*This is a medical classification.

If you are eighteen or less, however, the CDC uses different methods to assess BMI. You can check out your BMI at apps.nccd.cdc.gov/dnpabmi/calculator. aspx.

Types of Anorexia

Though many people only think of anorexia as the severe restriction of food, the disease is divided into two categories, the more familiar restricting form and binge-eating/purging.

Restricting Anorexia

Restricting anorexia is the most common form of the disease. Individuals with this type of anorexia severely limit the number of calories they consume. They also use excessive exercise to lose weight.

Binge-Eating/Purging Anorexia

The binge-eating/purging form of anorexia is diagnosed when individuals eat during binges and then purge by using laxatives, diuretics, enemas, or self-induced vomiting.

Complications of Anorexia

The psychological and physical effects of anorexia are damaging, even life threatening. The individual with anorexia often becomes depressed or suffers from severe mood swings. Physically, the lack of nutrition can damage the heart, liver, and kidneys. To preserve the energy it has, the body slows down, causing blood pressure, pulse, and breathing rates to drop. *Anemia*, swollen joints, and brittle bones can also develop in people with anorexia.

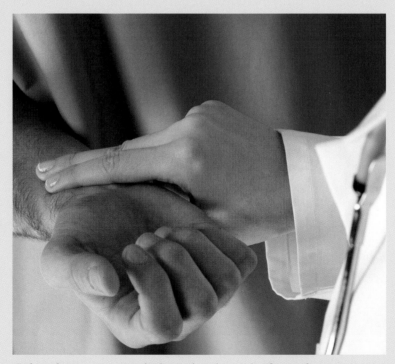

Other than severe weight loss, the physical effects of anorexia can include a slowed pulse and breathing rate.

The idea and process of losing weight consume the life of someone with anorexia. Physical and psychological health suffers, but so does the person's social life. Just think about how much time we spend eating with friends—whether lunch in the school cafeteria, popcorn at a movie, or a pizza after shopping at the mall. How many times can excuses like "I just ate," or "We're having a big dinner later," or "I have to study," or "I have to go for a run" be used before friends catch on? After a while, some individuals with anorexia find it easier to withdraw from friends than to come up with excuses.

The once-good student may now have difficulty concentrating, and schoolwork may suffer. The athlete or dancer who began dieting to enhance performance may find she is no longer competitive.

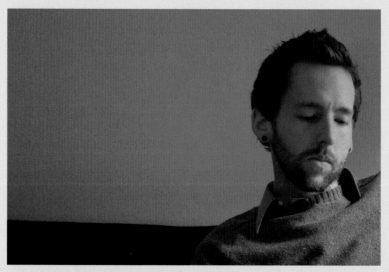

An individual with anorexia may stop going out with friends because he has run out of excuses for not eating.

Secrecy is a large part of being anorexic. Food and eating can become a well-planned ritual for the person with anorexia. She may sit down to meals with family members and push the food around the plate, trying to make it appear as though she's eaten something. Sometimes she will actually eat, but only small amounts of one particular food. People with anorexia can become obsessed with weighing not only themselves but also every bit of food they consume. Fat grams and carbohydrates are *meticulously* calculated. Others refuse to eat in front of people. Some with anorexia love cooking for friends and family members, but will not eat any of the meal themselves.

Bulimia Nervosa

Unlike the person with anorexia, who severely limits the amount of food she takes in, the person with bulimia regularly eats large amounts of food in a short period of time, much more than an average person would eat within the same time frame and situation. It is not unusual for individuals to eat and drink between 5,000 and 10,000 calories in a matter of minutes or hours.

In most cases, the person with bulimia then purges by using laxatives, enemas, diuretics, self-induced vomiting, or excessive exercise. Bulimia is the most common eating disorder; according to a 2006 report by the American Psychiatric Association, between 1.1 percent and 4.2 percent of females will have a period of bulimia at some point during their lifetime. According to the Canadian Mental Health Association, more than 114,000 women have bulimia in Canada.

Like most eating disorders, bulimia usually begins in adolescence, although it can appear at other times as well. Far more women than men are diagnosed with the disease. Bulimia is diagnosed more often in Caucasian women in Western countries.

The National Institute of Mental Health lists the following as the most common characteristics of bulimia:

1. Recurrent episodes of binge eating, characterized by eating an excessive amount of food

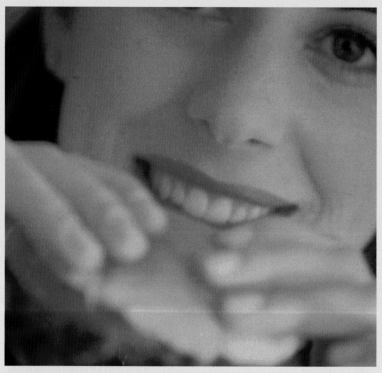

Bulimia is characterized by periods during which the individual binges, consuming as many as 10,000 calories in a very short amount of time.

within a discrete period of time and by a sense of lack of control over eating during the epi-sode

2. Recurrent inappropriate **compensatory** behav-ior in order to prevent weight gain, such as self-induced vomiting or misuse of laxatives, diuretics, enemas, or other medications (purg-ing); fasting; or excessive exercise

3. The binge eating and inappropriate compensa-tory behaviors both occur, on average, at least twice a week for three months

4. Self-evaluation is unduly influenced by body shape and weight

Bulimic behaviors are generally conducted in private.

Warning Signs of Bulimia

- throwing up after meals
- running water in the bathroom for long periods (to cover the sound of vomiting)
- overexercising
- calluses or scars on the knuckles from forced vomiting
- denial of an eating problem

Types of Bulimia

Like anorexia, bulimia is divided into two categories, purging and nonpurging.

Purging Bulimia

This is the most common form of bulimia. Someone with this form may use laxatives, diuretics, enemas, and most often self-induced vomiting to rid the body of calories consumed during the bingeing cycle. According to the National Institute of Mental Health, up to 90 percent of people with bulimia use self-induced vomiting to purge. Most often the fingers are used to induce vomiting, though items such as butter knives are sometimes used, especially in the beginning. The longer the habit of self-induced vomiting is practiced, the easier it will become for the person to vomit at will.

Nonpurging Bulimia

Someone diagnosed with nonpurging bulimia uses other methods to compensate for bingeing behaviors. Instead of vomiting or abusing laxatives and other medications, the person with this form of bulimia may skip meals or over-exercise to rid the body of the calories consumed during bingeing episodes.

Fast Fact

According to the National Institute of Mental Health, *over half of individuals diagnosed with anorexia will eventually develop bulimia.*

Complications of Bulimia

As with other eating disorders, bulimia has physical and psychological complications. Among the physical complications are fluid, **electrolyte**, and mineral imbalances (which can lead to problems in heart rhythm and **dehydration**) and menstrual irregularities including missed periods.

Many of the physical complications come from purging. These include the loss of tooth enamel, tooth decay, sore throat, kidney damage, **esophageal** tear, and stomach rupture. Though the latter two are rare, they are life threatening. Many individuals with bulimia suffer from almost constant stomach pain from vomiting.

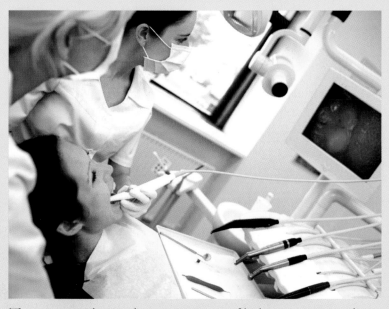

The vomiting during the purging stage of bulimia causes tooth decay and the loss of tooth enamel.

The abuse of laxatives may lead to a dependence on them as well as to rectal *prolapse* and *hemorrhoids*.

Sadly, food is not the only issue with which those with bulimia must deal. Many exhibit symptoms of depression and other mood disorders, often brought on by the isolation of the disease. According to the National Center on Addiction and Substance Abuse, alcohol, *methamphetamine*, cocaine, and heroin are used by some bulimics to increase *metabolism* and purge calories.

Perhaps the biggest complication of bulimia is the secrecy surrounding its practice. Unlike anorexia in which the self-induced starvation soon becomes apparent, someone with bulimia can hide the condition for years. The purging, dieting, and exercise that occur between binges helps the individual

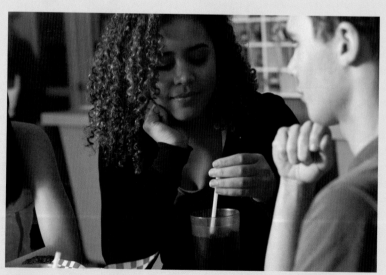

Unlike someone with anorexia, an individual with bulimia can keep her illness a secret because her weight may be within the normal range.

maintain a weight within or even slightly above the normal range. As with the person with anorexia, the individual with bulimia often isolates herself from friends and family. Although she might find it easier to eat with her friends, she still must have the privacy to perform purging behaviors.

Binge-Eating Disorder

Most of us know what it's like to eat more than usual. How many of us have actually left the Thanksgiving Day table still hungry? Or what about the restaurant buffet? We want to make sure we get our money's worth, after all!

To most people, such binges are an occasional occurrence. But for the approximately four million Americans with binge-eating disorder (also called compulsive overeating), it's not something that happens on special occasions. For them, bingeing is the "norm." Binge eating is the most prevalent eating disorder in America.

Symptoms of binge eating include:

- Recurrent episodes of binge eating, characterized by eating an excessive amount of food within a discrete period of time and by a sense of lack of control over eating during the episode.

- The binge-eating episodes are associated with at least three of the following: eating much more rapidly than normal; eating until feeling uncomfortably full; eating large amounts of food when not feeling physically hungry; eating alone because of being embarrassed by how much one is eating; feeling disgusted with oneself, depressed, or very guilty after overeating.

- Marked distress about binge-eating behavior.

- The binge eating occurs, on average, at least two days a week for six months.

- The binge eating is not associated with the regular use of inappropriate compensatory behaviors (i.e., purging, fasting, excessive exercise).

Binge-eating disorder can mirror bulimia except in one important way. People with this disorder do not purge their bodies of the food. They may fast periodically or go on repetitive diets, but they do not abuse laxatives, diuretics, or exercise.

As with other eating disorders, binge eating is most common among women, but the difference is slight; for every three women with binge-eating disorder, two men have it. According to some experts, it is the most common eating disorder among men. Unlike anorexia and bulimia, binge eating occurs equally among black and white people. Although some teens have the disorder, it is found most often in adults between ages forty-six and fifty-five.

Binge Eating, Diets, and Other Potential Causes

As with anorexia and bulimia, scientists aren't sure what causes binge-eating disorder. There is an unclear relationship between dieting and this

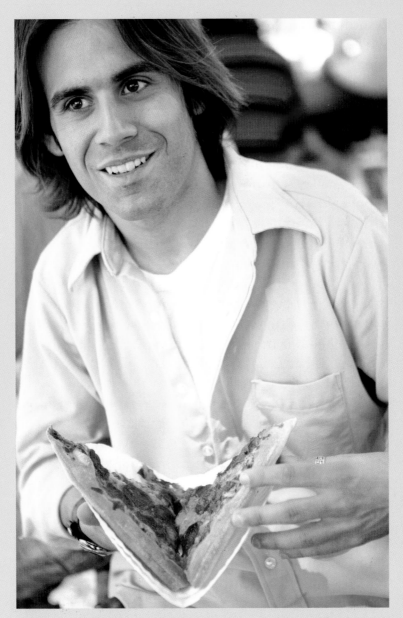

Binge eating disorder involves eating vast quantities of food in a short amount of time, but without the purging episodes of bulimia.

disorder. Approximately 10 to 15 percent of people who are slightly obese and try to lose the weight on their own through the use of commercial weight-loss programs are diagnosed with binge-eating disorder. Studies have shown that approximately 50 percent of individuals with the disorder had episodes prior to dieting. Some people binge eat after dieting. Many doctors recommend that people with binge-eating disorder who are not overweight—and not all are—should not skip meals, drastically reduce the amount of food eaten daily, or restrict certain types of foods (carbohydrates, for example), as these behaviors can make the disorder worse.

According to some studies, as many as 50 percent of those with binge-eating disorders report a history of depression. However, which came first isn't clear—did the depression cause the disorder, or did the disorder cause the depression? Or are both genetically linked?

Many people with the disorder report that feelings of anger, sadness, boredom, and worry can send them into a binge-eating episode. Many of us curl up with a bowl of ice cream or other comfort food when feeling sad, and this is fine—once in a while. But for the person with binge-eating disorder, this happens much more often. Impulse-control disorders also tend to be common among people with binge-eating disorder.

Researchers are also looking at how the body's metabolism affects the disorder. Other researchers are working with the **hypothesis** that there is a genetic connection to binge-eating disorders; several members of a family often have the disorder.

Complications of Binge-Eating Disorder

The most obvious complications of binge-eating disorder are those related to excessive weight. Some people with binge-eating disorder are not overweight or obese, but most are. People with the disorder also tend to become overweight at a younger age.

The weight gain that can come with binge-eating disorder, and the obesity that can follow, can lead to:

- type-2 diabetes (formerly called adult-onset diabetes)
- high blood pressure
- high cholesterol levels
- gallbladder disease
- heart disease
- *musculoskeletal* disorders
- certain cancers

Some studies have found that in general, people with binge-eating disorder report more health problems, stress, sleep disorders, and suicidal thoughts than do people without an eating disorder. For many, feelings of self-hatred and disgust fill their thoughts. Feelings of shame can drive people with binge-eating disorder to a life of isolation.

Eating disorders are serious illnesses. According to the Web site Focus Adolescent Services, without treatment, 20 percent of people with an eating disorder will die. With treatment, the death rate falls to 2 to 3 percent.

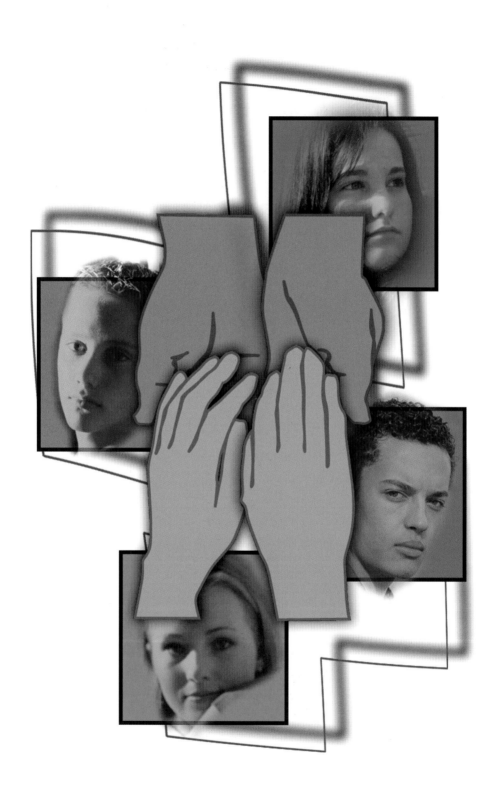

Chapter 3
Finally Popular?

On a Saturday morning a few weeks later, Susan stared at the computer. Picking a subject for Mr. Paulson's paper had been more difficult than she had thought it would be. After giving it a lot of thought, she hit on the perfect topic—thinness, or rather, how different societies' idea of perfect body size has changed throughout history. Susan had written a detailed outline and research plan and presented it to Mr. Paulson.

"Susan, this is really interesting," Mr. Paulson had told her. "Go for it."

That was three weeks ago, and that's as far as Susan had gotten on her paper, due on Monday. It was crunch time, and Susan knew it. She was sure that Gina, Anne, and practically every other teen in town had slept in that morning, but she had gotten up at 6:00. Now, as she heard the clock downstairs chime noon, she sat waiting for words to pop up on her computer. Susan had always liked doing research, but actually putting words down on paper—or on the computer screen—had always been much more difficult for her. *Oh well, I'll do some more research*, Susan thought, stalling the inevitable.

Then, she caught a glimpse of something out of the corner of her eye. Susan picked up a pencil and poked at it, pushing it a little to the left, then a little to the right. Finally, she used the pencil's eraser to drag the bag of chips closer to her. "Oh well, what can it hurt?" she asked aloud as she ripped open the package and snarfed down the snack. She licked the salt off her lips and smiled. It had been a long time since she'd had chips.

"Susan, phone."

Her mother's voice calling from downstairs was a not-so-welcome interruption. Susan had finally gotten momentum going, and her paper was coming along nicely. "Mom, can you take a message?"

"Okay, but it's that Brooke person again."

"Got it, Mom. Thanks." Susan picked up the phone. "Hi, Brooke."

"Hey, Susan. Watcha doin'? Jessica, Syd, and I are going to a movie. Wanna come?"

Susan couldn't believe her ears. She had pretty much given up on being friends with Brooke and her crowd. Since the "dieting lesson" in the library, Brooke hadn't made any effort to talk to Susan. And other than slipping Susan the cryptic thank-you note in the coffee shop, Brooke hadn't even acknowledged that she existed. Now, here at last was another chance to be popular. "Sure," Susan replied, trying not to sound too excited (or desperate). "That sounds great!"

"Cool. We'll pick you up around seven. Okay? That's Penrose Avenue, right?"

Susan confirmed her address and hung up the phone. "I've worked enough today," she said as she shut off the computer and went to her closet to pick out an outfit. She was so glad that she now had several fashionable outfits from which to choose.

She heard the phone ring again, and for the second time in just a few minutes, her mother called up the stairs, "Susan, phone."

"Hi, Suz," Gina's familiar voice came through the receiver. "Do you want to do something tonight?"

Well, now. This is quite a quandary. Susan quickly searched for an answer, one that wouldn't hurt her friend's feelings. "Oh, I'm sorry, Gina. I already have something to do. It's not a biggie. Maybe we can do something tomorrow."

"That's all right. I know it's last minute and all. I just thought you might be free. Annie's doing some family thing."

As Susan hung up the phone, she thought about what Gina—her friend—had said. *How dare she assume that I'd be free! I have new friends, popular ones even.*

Dressed in jeans and a cute top she was sure she'd never worn to school, Susan bounded down the stairs to wait for the girls. "You know, Mom," she said as she joined her mother in the living room, "maybe I should have my own cell phone. A lot of the girls do you know."

"Well, I *don't* know that, but we'll see, Susan, we'll see," her mother answered. Susan didn't think her own phone sounded too promising.

A horn beeped outside, and Susan told her mother good-bye and went to meet her friends.

"Hi, Susan," greeted Brooke as Susan joined Sydney in the backseat. Susan told Sydney and Jessica hello as the car pulled out onto the street. Sydney, Jessica, and Brooke seemed to pick up on whatever they had been talking about before Susan joined them. Their inside jokes and laughing made Susan feel out of place on the ride to the theater. *I'm just lucky to be included,* she kept reminding herself.

As the girls waited at the snack counter, Susan had a chance to take a look at Brooke. She seemed thinner—a lot thinner. Susan knew that she hadn't really seen Brooke much in the past few weeks, but she couldn't believe how much weight she seemed to have lost. *I guess if you're thin to begin with,* Susan rationalized, *any weight you lose seems exaggerated.* Sydney and Jessica didn't seem too concerned. "Popcorn, ladies?" asked the guy behind the counter. Brooke didn't ask anyone what they wanted, just told the guy they'd be sharing the largest tub of popcorn, but that she wanted a large box of chocolate mints as well.

Susan didn't really care for the movie. She wasn't a big fan of Leonardo DiCaprio, but she was content to be there with her new friends. She looked down the row, and everyone seemed to be having a good time. The tub of popcorn was passed from girl to girl, but toward the end of the movie, Susan noticed that she seemed to have it more than the others. Still, she tried to limit how much popcorn she ate.

"I have to stop in the ladies' room," Brooke announced as the girls were leaving the movie theater.

"We'll wait here," Jessica said, and she, Sydney, and Susan moved out of the way of the other moviegoers.

"So, Susan, what did you think of the movie?" asked Sydney. Susan was never any good at small talk, but she wanted to be Sydney's friend, too. The fact that Sydney wasn't looking at her when she asked Susan about the movie didn't do much to make her feel comfortable, though. *Okay, this is my first night out with these guys. Don't muck it up!*

"It was pretty good. What did you think?"

"I liked it a lot," piped up Jessica. "I just love Leonardo."

"Me too," said Sydney. "What's not to like?"

Susan just nodded. *Now what do I say? I wish Brooke would get back. I don't have anything to say to these girls.* "I wonder what's taking Brooke so long. Do you think we should check on her?"

Sydney and Jessica snickered. "No," reassured Jessica, "I'm sure she's all right. Sometimes she just takes a little while in the bathroom."

Finally, after what seemed to Susan to be an incredibly long time, Brooke rejoined the girls.

"So, is everyone up for a trip to the coffee shop? Scott and the guys should be there." Brooke led her troops to the car.

Wow! Now everyone will see me—Susan—at the coffee shop with the in crowd! I have arrived.

The coffee shop wasn't very crowded when the girls arrived, but the "usuals" were there at their usual tables. Brooke had been right: Scott, Jeff, and Paul were there waiting for them. *Oh no, I'm a third wheel,* thought Susan. "Hi, ladies," Scott greeted the girls.

"Hi, Susan, I'm glad you made it." At first, Susan couldn't tell who had made a point of speaking to her, but then she saw him—Nick Murphy. Like the other guys, he was a senior and a jock; he was on the basketball and track teams.

"Like our surprise, Susan?" smiled Brooke. Then it hit her. This was a set-up. Brooke wanted her to have a boyfriend—one from their crowd. And, well, she had to admit that Nick was very good looking.

"Who wouldn't?" laughed Susan.

The group sat down and ordered a pizza. The menu at the coffee shop was limited, but it was known for its killer pizzas.

In the shop's bright lights, Susan could get a better look at Brooke. *Brooke looks like she's been sick. And look at her wrists: they're so bony.*

"So, Susan, are you going to the dance next month?" asked Jessica. Susan could swear that she saw Nick blush at the question.

"I don't know. I'm pretty busy," Susan answered, hoping that the others wouldn't ask her what was keeping her so busy. In truth, she didn't have anything to do, and she would love to go to the dance. She had never gone to a high school dance. Fortunately, the pizza came just then, and it kept the six of them occupied.

All right, Susan, you can have one slice. You've eaten mostly junk today, but this is a special occasion.

Brooke, Jessica, and Sydney were dominating the conversation, so Susan was able to relax. She was surprised that she felt so comfortable here with people who were basically strangers. Susan felt so comfortable that it seemed completely natural for her to reach for a second, and then a third slice of pizza. *I really haven't had* that *much to eat today.* She noticed that she wasn't the only one enjoying the pizza. She and Brooke must have eaten half of the large pizza.

Too soon, the coffee shop manager told them he had to close. "Let me take a quick ladies' room pit stop and then I can take you home," Brooke told Susan and the other girls, "unless you want to take her home, Nick." Again Susan was sure that Nick had blushed.

"Uh, I'm sorry, Susan. I-I-I didn't drive."

"That's all right, Nick. I can wait for Brooke."
The guys left, and once again Susan, Jessica, and Sydney were waiting for Brooke.

"Are you sure Brooke is all right? Maybe we should go in and make sure." Susan was getting a bad feeling about things and was ready to go check on Brooke when Sydney grabbed her arm.

"No," Sydney told Susan, "Brooke is fine. She just needs some privacy. Let's wait for her outside."

The three walked outside. At the end of the parking lot, Susan saw the guys getting into Scott's car. Well, all except one. Nick was getting into the driver's seat of another car. He had lied to her.

"Okay, ladies. Off we go." Brooke came bouncing out the coffee shop door. As they piled into her car, Susan suddenly couldn't wait to get home. Her perfect evening had been ruined.

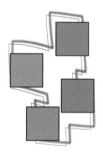

Who Develops Eating Disorders?

No one knows exactly what causes someone to develop an eating disorder. Two facts are known: eating disorders occur mostly in girls and women, and most eating disorders develop during adolescence, although the initial age of diagnosis is lowering.

Personality

Although everyone is unique, there are certain personality traits common to most people with an eating disorder:

- low self-esteem
- feelings of helplessness
- a fear of becoming fat

Stress, including the stress to be thin, also seems to play an important part in the development of eating disorders. Many believe that people with anorexia use their denial of food as a way to gain control of their lives. They are often *perfectionists*, good students and athletes who seldom disobey the authority figures in their lives. Their concern for pleasing others means that they may not have developed the coping skills necessary for dealing with the issues of adolescence. However, they can control their food intake and their weight.

Individuals with bulimia and those who binge eat often eat large amounts of food to cope with stress and other issues such as loneliness.

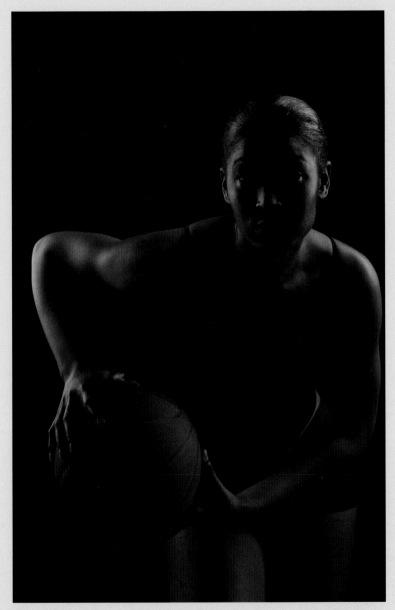

People who develop eating disorders are often good students or athletes who tend to be perfectionists.

Genetics and the Environment

As with many psychiatric and medical conditions, there appears to be a *familial* component to the development of eating disorders, usually among the female members of a family. Genetics and the environment play a role in the development of eating disorders. Some studies indicate that girls with mothers overly concerned with their daughters' weight and girls with fathers and brothers who are very critical of their weight are more likely to develop an eating disorder. A parent who is overly concerned with her own appearance also models that behavior to her children, increasing the likelihood that they will have the same exaggerated concern with their

Fast Fact

- At least 8 million people in the United States have an eating disorder.
- Ninety percent of those with an eating disorder are women.
- People with eating disorders may be rich or poor, although it is more common among higher income groups.
- Eating disorders usually start in the teens but may begin as early as age eight.

own bodies. In many cases, this leads to an eating disorder.

Biochemical

The *neuroendocrine system* is the body's regulatory mechanism. Working together, the central nervous system and the hormone system control such functions as growth and development, appetite and digestion, sleep, and emotions. One or more of these areas is

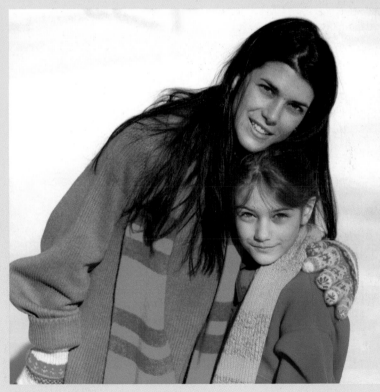

Eating disorders seem to run in families. However, it is more likely learned behavior than genetics.

often working improperly in someone with an eating disorder.

Neurotransmitters control hormone production in the brain. Researchers discovered decreased amounts of two neurotransmitters—serotonin and norepinephrine—in the brain chemistry of individuals with anorexia and bulimia, and with depression and other mood disorders. It is unclear if the low levels of neurotransmitters cause eating disorders, or if eating

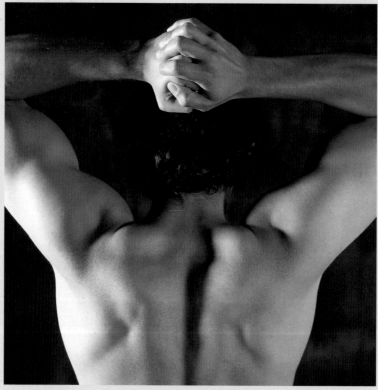

Though eating disorders occur more often in women, men also suffer from trying to attain the media image of the perfect male body.

disorders create the abnormal brain chemistry, but researchers hope that using treatments developed for those conditions may help people living with an eating disorder.

Eating Disorders and Men

From what one sees in the media, you might think only women have eating disorders. While it is true that most individuals with eating disorders are women, an estimated 10 percent are men. Most of the men with an eating disorder have either bulimia or binge-eating disorder.

The causes of eating disorders in men do not differ from those that cause them in women. Stress affects men, too, and the media has its own view of what makes a man attractive. It might be more obvious when men develop an eating disorder as an emotional response to a problem.

For the most part, treatment methods for men with eating disorders do not differ greatly than those for women. However, men may find the process more difficult. Men often have a more difficult time admitting they have a health problem, which can delay the seeking of treatment. Then there is the awkwardness that men might feel when participating in a group therapy session populated mostly by women. However, for both men and women, eating disorders are serious illnesses that need to be addressed by professionals.

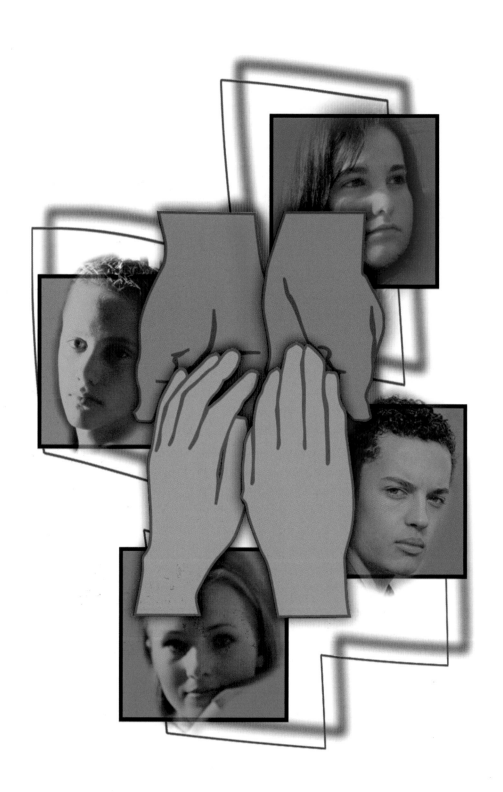

Chapter 4
Coming Clean

"O h man," whined Susan, "I must have PMS water weight gain. Someday I'm going to invent a cure for that. I'll get rich!"

She struggled to fasten the zipper on a pair of pants that had fit perfectly just a few weeks before. She, Anne, and Gina were in her room, along with a big bag of chips and sodas. Anne and Gina glanced at each other; Susan saw Anne shrug her shoulders and mouth, "You tell her."

"Well, Susan," Gina started, "you know we love you, so, well, Anne and I have noticed that you've been eating more like you did before you went to camp."

Anne chimed in with agreement. "That's right, sweetie. We didn't want to say anything, because you know how we feel about you doesn't have anything to do with weight. But Suz, you'd been doing so well. What happened, honey?"

Susan gave up trying to fasten her pants and dropped onto the bed beside Gina and Anne. *What had happened?* she wondered. "Nothing happened, that's what happened." Susan knew she was lying to her friends, but if *she* didn't know why she was eating so badly again, how could she explain it to these two, neither of whom had ever once had a weight problem. "I'm sure it's just PMS. Gina, you know how you get chocolate cravings. And Anne, don't you go nuts for salty food when you have PMS? Well, I'm just eating a little more for the same reason." *They sure can't argue about that!*

"That makes sense, Suz," said Anne, and Gina nodded in agreement. She also pulled a chocolate bar out of her pocket and tossed it into Susan's trashcan, causing the other girls to erupt in giggles. *This seems so normal, so right.*

Changing the subject, Anne asked, "So, how did you do on Paulson's paper? It was keeping you so busy for quite a while."

Susan felt more than a little guilty. Yes, the paper had kept her busy, but not busy enough to stop her from going out with Brooke. Actually, her new plan hadn't really worked at all. Just like most of her other papers, she hadn't finished it until the night before it was due. Still, Mr. Paulson had given her an "A." "I got an 'A' on it, but I think it was because the subject was different from what others were writing about. I don't think it was my best work."

Gina rolled over on the bed, "Oh Suz, you're just too hard on yourself. Congrats."

Changing the subject, Anne asked, "Suz, do you want to go to a movie or something? How about the coffee shop?" Anne and Gina had asked her to go to the coffee shop with them several times lately, but Susan had turned them down each time. Coming up with believable excuses was getting incredibly difficult. Susan hadn't wanted to go back since the night she'd been there with Brooke and the others. Part of her was relieved that Brooke hadn't invited her out since that night two weeks ago. Susan knew that Sydney and Jessica knew that Nick had lied to her about the car. She was just as sure that they had told Brooke. At school, Susan had made a point of avoiding places where she might run into Brooke. Since she wasn't a cheerleader or dating an athlete, she had found that to be amazingly easy.

But it was time to end her exile. "Sure, let's go to the coffee shop. I'm tired of being cooped up here. But let me find a pair of pants that fit first!"

It was early evening by the time the girls got to the coffee shop, and most of the tables were taken by couples out on dates. They found a table near the back, where they could sit and watch everyone come in. The girls ordered sodas (diet for Susan, who felt Gina and Anne watching) and salads. *You know, Gina and Anne really do have my best interests at heart. They could eat anything, but they're having salad.* Just as the food arrived, the door opened and familiar laughing came into the coffee shop. Brooke, Jessica, and Sydney came in along with their boyfriends; they were part of the coffee shops "usuals." *Don't let them see me,* Susan pleaded internally, but it was useless. "Susan!" Brooke called just a little too loudly. She hurried over to the table. "It seems like ages since we went out. Let's make plans to go out next weekend, okay?" Susan nodded, hoping Brooke would leave. "Great! Oh, hi, uh . . ."

"Gina and Anne," Susan quickly prompted. Brooke gave a quick little wave and hurried off to join the others.

Gina and Anne looked at each other, and then at Susan. "You went out with prom queen and her court?" Gina asked.

"Just once," Susan admitted. "It was no big deal. We just went to a movie. Then we came here for pizza."

Anne laughed. "Sheez, Susan, you act as though you cheated on us."

"Yeah, Suz. We're friends, not dates," laughed Gina.

"You're not mad?" Susan had been afraid to tell them about it. She was sure that she would have been angry in their places.

Anne and Gina shook their heads. "Why would we be?" Gina asked.

"Did you stand us up to go out with them," Anne wanted to know.

"Oh, I'd never do that. Gina, it was that night you called and wanted to know if I wanted to do something. Anne had family plans or something." Gina nodded. "Brooke had already asked me to go to the movies with her, Sydney, and Jessica."

"Did you have a good time?" Gina asked.

"I did at first, but it didn't end so hot." Susan told her friends about coming to the coffee shop—and Nick.

"Well," said Anne, "all I can say is that it's his loss." She raised her glass of soda, and Susan, Gina, and Anne clinked their glasses in agreement.

It's been a long time since I've felt this good, thought Susan.

The girls enjoyed their salad—and each other's company. But Susan couldn't help looking over at Brooke's table. She was kind of envious of the laughing—and the large pizza—the group was sharing. Still, there was something about Brooke. For some reason, Susan had a hard time keeping her eyes off of her, though at the same time, it was incredibly hard to look at her. Apparently, Anne and Gina had the same problem, though each tried to keep it from the others.

Finally, Gina leaned over and whispered, "Suz, is there something wrong with Brooke?"

Susan shrugged her shoulders. Brooke looked even worse than she had just a couple of weeks ago. Her eyes were sunken deep into their sockets, and her blouse seemed to hang shapelessly on her shoulders. Still, she and the others were laughing and joking around. "I don't know," Susan sighed. *But I'm beginning to have my suspicions.*

Later that night, Susan went online and Googled eating disorders.

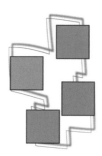

How Do You Tell If Someone Has an Eating Disorder?

It is not unusual to be concerned about weight and appearance. However, if a friend has any of the following signs, it may indicate that he or she has an eating disorder:

- an obsession with food, such as counting every calorie or fat gram eaten
- avoids foods he or she used to love.
- exercises too much although thin and losing weight
- becomes less social and more competitive in school, sports, and other activities
- doesn't feel as though he or she is good enough in anything
- never lets you see what he or she is eating
- continues to lose weight even though thin
- wears large, oversized clothes though thin
- uses diet pills, water pills, or laxatives
- throws up after eating
- smokes a lot to lost weight
- has fainting spells
- has not started her menstrual period though most her age have, or if she had started her period, stopped for no known reason

(Adapted from Canadian Health Network, http://www.canadian-health-network.ca, August 2004.)

Physical signs of anorexia or bulimia include:
- noticeable weight loss, especially in anorexia
- throat irritation caused by repeated vomiting
- growth of fine body hair
- excessive constipation
- swollen lymph and salivary glands

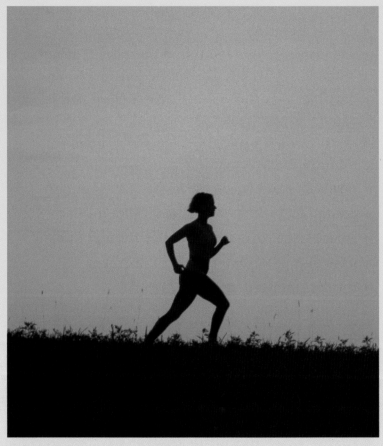

If a friend seems to be exercising a lot even though she is very thin, it might be a sign she has an eating disorder.

- depression and mood swings
- menstrual irregularities and cessation
- tooth loss and decay
- heart irregularities
- hyperactivity
- dry skin
- dizziness
- puffy face
- yellowish tint to skin
- cold, mottled hands and feet
- thinning of hair on head, dry and brittle hair
- feeling cold all of the time

If You Think Your Friend Has an Eating Disorder

1. Tell your friend that you are concerned and care about his or her well-being.

2. Encourage him or her to talk to a counselor or therapist. Remember, you are a friend, not a trained therapist.

3. Try to get your friend to discuss how he or she feels.

4. Get support from an adult you trust and educate yourself.

5. Be positive! People do recover from eating disorders.

What Not to Do

1. Don't focus on weight, food, or exercise. Remember, these are symptoms of the problem, not the problem.

2. Do not lay on guilt trips. Your friend feels bad enough already.

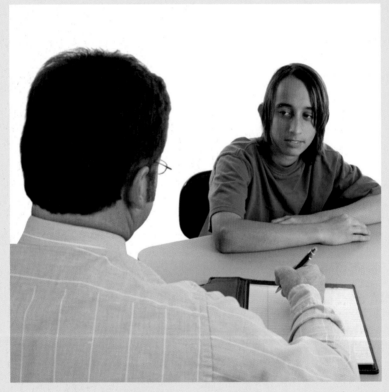

If you are worried about a friend's eating habits, encourage him to talk to a counselor or therapist.

3. Do not treat your friend as though he or she has a disability. Treat your friend as normally as possible. It'll help.

4. Don't be afraid to discuss conflicts or problems.

5. Don't blame yourself. Friends don't cause eating disorders, but they can help in the recovery process.

6. Don't focus on the amount of weight gained or lost. Focus more on your friend's mental state than on his or her physical state.

7. Don't focus on achievements—grades, sporting events, and promotions. Talk about inner qualities and strengths. Also talk about your own failures and mistakes.

(Source: MEDA, www.medainc.org)

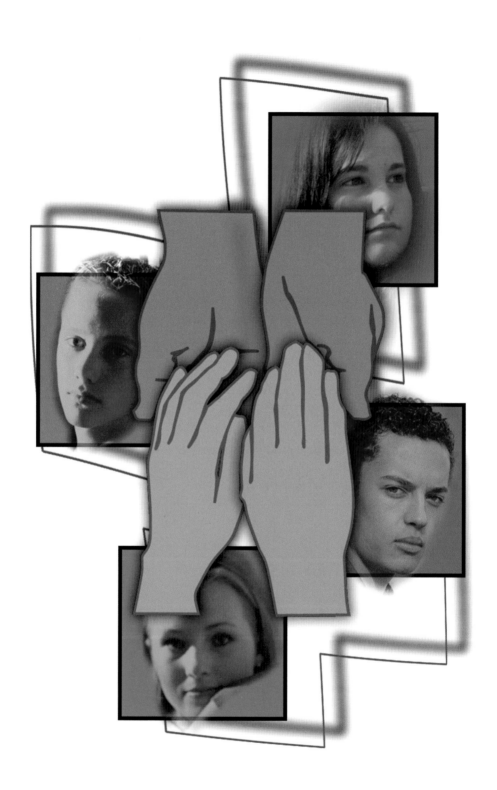

Chapter 5
Calling the Cavalry

Susan!" Gina yelled into the phone.

"Gina," Susan calmly and quietly replied, "we're not talking on a tin-can phone. You don't have to yell."

"Sorry. Did you hear what happened after we left the coffee shop?"

"No. I've been trying to catch up on homework all day. What happened, for crying out loud."

"They had to call an ambulance to take Brooke to the hospital! She fainted or something. I knew there had to be something wrong with that girl. She looked like she'd break if you touched her. Are you sure you don't know what's wrong with her?"

"No, not really. Uh, Gina, I have to go, all right?"

"Sure, I've got to call and tell Anne. Talk to you later. Bye."

Ah, thought Susan, *the information superhighway had nothing on Gina when it came to getting out information.*

Susan had spent a lot of time on the computer after she got home from the coffee shop the night before. When she was doing research for her paper for Mr. Paulson's class, she'd come across information on eating disorders. She'd found that many experts believe eating disorders are perhaps caused—or at least worsened—by a society's emphasis on being thin. At least today's Western society. She had been kind of surprised that some cultures had actually preferred a rounder figure. *Oh to have those days back*, she laughed to herself.

Of course Susan had learned something about eating disorders at camp during the previous summer. The campers, however, were like her; they had problems with eating too much. They all *knew* they were fat; there was no way around that. Still, Brenna had talked about bulimia, because some overweight people also suffer from bulimia or even anorexia. And some overweight people had another eating disorder, Brenna had said, called binge eating. *If I were going to have an eating disorder, that's the one I'd probably have*, Susan thought ruefully.

Last night, as Susan had looked up more details on bulimia and anorexia, she recalled Brooke's lengthy trips to the bathroom after going to the movie and having pizza at the coffee shop. Neither Jessica nor Sydney had seemed alarmed. *Hmm. I wonder if all of them have bulimia.* According to the information she read, it would not have been that unusual for a group of friends to all have an eating disorder. They all ate a lot that night. Susan tried to remember what Brooke had eaten when she'd seen her at the coffee shop at other times. It always seemed that the table was getting a large pizza, but pizza is a staple of the teenage diet, after all.

Then Susan remembered the conversation she had with Brooke in the library just after school started that year. Brooke had asked her how she'd lost weight, and Brooke was concerned that she herself was getting too fat. *That's right. She was really disappointed to find out that there was nothing magic about how I lost weight. Just eating right and exercise.* Then there was that note Brooke had left on her table at the coffee shop. Brooke had written that she'd found a solution. Susan was certain that she didn't know Brooke well enough to be able to tell what exactly that solution was, but after seeing her at the coffee shop, she was sure that at least part of Brooke's solution to her weight problem was an eating disorder.

That was last night, and now Susan was sure that it was an eating disorder that had sent Brooke to the hospital. A soft knock on her door brought Susan out of her deep thoughts.

"Susan," her mother said as she opened the door, "Could we talk?"

"Sure." Susan turned to face her mother as she sat on the edge of the bed.

"Susan," her mother started hesitantly, "I just heard about Brooke. Isn't she the one you went to the movie with a few weeks ago?" Susan nodded. "I ran into Gina's mother at the grocery store," Susan's mother continued, "and she said that Brooke had to be taken to the hospital. Did you hear about that?"

"Gina called a few minutes ago and told me. Mom, we saw Brooke at the coffee shop last night, and she looked terrible. I think she has an eating disorder."

"You might be right. Gina's mother told me that she heard Brooke was in pretty bad shape, something about electrolytes and her organs not functioning right."

"If the eating disorder is serious enough, the kidneys can shut down. Mom, people die from eating disorders."

Susan's mother nodded. "Susan, honey, can we talk about you now?"

"Me? I don't have bulimia or anorexia. And I'm not a compulsive eater."

"Susan, don't get so defensive. I'm not saying you have an eating disorder like Brooke might have. I've just noticed a few things, and I'd like us to talk about them." Susan tried to relax, but her stomach was tied in knots waiting to hear what her mother had to say. "Susan, you know I love you and will love you no matter what. That's just a fact that will never change. Now, having said that, I admit that I was very happy that you decided to go to camp last summer to get your weight under control. It has absolutely nothing to do with how you look; I just want you to be healthy. I was so proud when you came home. You were on your way to having your weight under control. You had really come a long way in learning about nutrition and how to select a balanced diet. And you weren't waiting at the door when I got home from the store, waiting to see what kind of chips or cookies I had bought." Her mother laughed.

That's true, Susan thought, *chips and cookies don't seem that important anymore.* "I did learn a lot at camp, Mom." Susan struggled to be honest, not only with her mother but with herself. She hadn't wanted to admit that she was eating again the way she always had. "I tried to keep with it, I really did."

"Oh honey, I know." Susan's mom reached over to take her daughter's hand. "I know you might find this hard to believe, but I do know that it's hard to deal with a weight problem. When I was your age, I had problems, too, but I worked at getting my eating habits under control—just like you did."

Susan took a look at her mom, finding it hard to believe that she had ever had a problem with her weight. "But you're thin. I don't remember you ever being heavy."

"That was long before you were born. But I had a problem, and I dealt with it. I have been so proud of how you've been handling your issues with weight. But we both know that, well, you've had some problems sticking to the plan lately. Right?"

Susan began to cry.

Her mother's hand tightened around hers. "Honey, don't cry. It'll be all right. Why don't you send Brenna an e-mail?"

Brenna! Why hadn't she thought of that?

Brenna,
Hi. This is Susan Madison. I was at camp this past summer. You told us that we could contact you if we had any questions or problems. Well, I'm having kind of a problem. Do you think we could meet and talk?
Thanks,
Susan

Susan decided she'd spent too much time in her room, so she decided to go for a walk. *At least that's a step in the right direction—no pun intended.* She walked to the flower shop on Grand Avenue and bought her mom some flowers. *Mom really has been great. Some mothers are all caught up on appearance, but Mom isn't. She's always putting me and my feelings first.* The hospital wasn't far from the flower shop, and Susan momentarily thought about stopping to see Brooke. But they weren't really friends, and besides, Susan wasn't sure what she could say to her.

When Susan checked her e-mail after she got home, she was happy to find an answer from Brenna:

> Susan,
> Hi! Of course I remember you. I'm sorry you're having some problems. How about if we meet tomorrow morning? The café on the Promenade? Unless I hear otherwise from you, I'll meet you there at 10:00.
> Hope to see you,
> Brenna

Ten tomorrow morning. Susan could hardly wait.

Susan left for the Promenade earlier than was really necessary, but she didn't want to take the chance that Brenna would get there first and think she wasn't coming. At ten sharp, Brenna came up to Susan's table.

"Susan, I'm so glad to see you. How about something to drink? Do you want anything to eat?" Susan hesitated, and Brenna smiled. "Susan, it's all right to drink and to eat. Actually, the fact of the matter is that both are necessary." Susan smiled back and ordered a coffee and bagel with cream cheese. She was relieved when Brenna did the same.

"Okay, Susan. What's up?"

Susan wasn't sure where she should begin. "Well, I've kind of gotten off track. I'm eating chips, cookies, huge amounts of pizza, ice cream, sodas, I'm not exercising like I should . . ."

"Whoa, Susan. Not so fast. All right, you're eating things that you know you probably shouldn't and you're eating more than you know you should. Do you know why?"

"Uh, isn't that what you're supposed to tell me?"

Brenna laughed. "I can't tell you why you're doing those things. That's *your* job. Let's see if we can figure this out together. What did you expect when you came back from camp?"

"Well, I thought I'd have lots of new clothes. Hmm, I got those. I thought I'd do better in gym and not look so bad in those dorky uniforms. That happened. I knew I'd feel better, you know, have more energy and all. That sure happened."

Brenna smiled. "Was there anything else? Something you really wanted to happen but that didn't? You need to be honest about what expectations you had."

How did she know? Susan looked down at the table and answered very quietly. "I thought I'd be popular. You know, have a boyfriend and all. That didn't happen. Well, not really." Susan described her night out with Brooke, and then she told Brenna about Nick's lie. "I just want to eat like I used to sometimes. It makes me feel better."

Brenna put her hand on top of Susan's. "Susan, remember what I told everyone the last night of camp? Your physical appearance changed, and it will take time for others to get used to the new you. It will take time for you to get used to the new you. Don't rush things. When things don't go the way we want them to, it is very common for us to go back to behaviors that are familiar to us. For many of us, that means eating the way we used to."

"But how can we avoid doing that?"

"Well, for me, I write in a journal. When I'm feeling stressed or disappointed, I've learned to write in a journal instead of turn to two of my former best friends—Ben and Jerry." Susan laughed. She could relate; she had been very close friends of theirs as well. "Put your feelings into words. Discuss possible solutions or alternatives. And it doesn't have to be a 'diary.' Write stories or poetry. Expand your horizons."

"That could work," Susan said with an excitement she'd not felt in a while.

"But Susan," Brenna cautioned, "that doesn't mean you'll never again face disappointment or experience temptation to go back to old behaviors. Hey, it's normal to get off track every once in a while. The secret to long-term success is to get back on track."

"But, Brenna, now I feel like I have some hope—that I'm not doomed to being overweight. And, if I nip it in the bud now, I won't have so much weight to lose." Susan realized that she'd heard those words before—from Brooke. "Brenna, I know someone who is in the hospital, probably with an eating disorder. She asked me how I'd lost weight. I told her there wasn't a magic cure, and I think she developed an eating disorder."

"Stop right there, Susan. If your friend has an eating disorder, it's not your fault. There are probably as many reasons why people develop eating disorders as there are people with eating disorders. And I can assure you of one thing without fear of contradiction—you're not one of those causes."

"But what can I do to help?"

"Be a friend, be supportive. You know that your friend will have a long way to go, and she could probably use your help."

Susan nodded. She was ready to be a friend to Brooke— if she'd let her.

How to Help a Friend With an Eating Disorder

It is only natural to want to help a friend who has a problem. As much as you might want to help, you must keep in mind that there are things you cannot—or should not—do. For example:

- You can't make your friend eat properly.
- You can't make your friend go into counseling.
- You shouldn't monitor what your friend is eating.
- You can't solve your friend's problems.

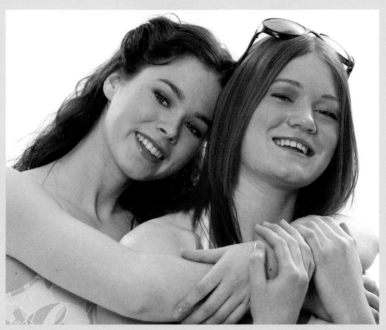

Support your friend, but remember you are not a trained expert.

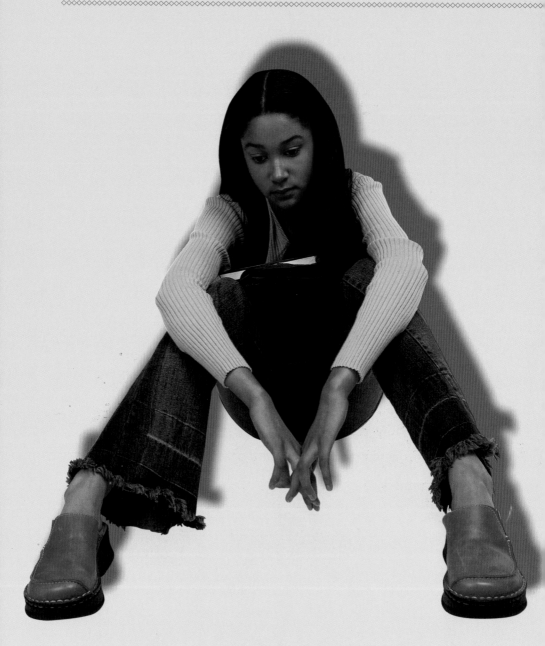

Eating disorders often develop when an individual feels too much stress in her life. Disordered eating becomes a way to control at least one aspect of her life.

What *can* you do?

- You can let your friend know you are there and that you care for him or her.

- You can discuss specific concerns you have about his or her health.

- You can be supportive of a friend in treatment.

- You can help your friend find support and treatment programs once he or she has decided to seek help.

Of course you want to **empathize** with your friend, but unless you've had an eating disorder, you do not know what she is going through or how she feels. Don't say things like "I skipped eating for three days, so I know how you feel," or "If I could throw up all the extra food I ate, it would make things so much better." No, you don't, and no, it doesn't.

Your friend's relationship with food is probably a symptom of another problem, one surrounding how he or she deals with stress and emotional issues. As stated on the Something Fishy Web site (www.something-fishy.org), "disordered eating is an attempt to control, to hide, stuff, avoid and forget emotional pain, stress and/or self-hate."

Are Eating Disorders Always Bad?

Yes they are—but according to some Web sites, having an eating disorder is a lifestyle choice. These pro–eating disorder (pro-ed), pro-anorexia (pro-ana), or pro-bulimia (pro-Mia) sites offer tips on how to eat less and lose more, how to purge, message boards to offer support and brag about the latest number of pounds lost, and photos. Ana and Mia are treated like real people. Teenage girls and young women, those most likely to have an eating disorder, write most of the sites.

According to a Stanford University study, 40 percent of teens with an eating disorder visit a pro-ed site; only 34 percent visit sites that deal with overcoming such disorders. And the popularity of pro–eating disorder sites is growing. A Google search in December 2005 of the key word pro-anorexia produced 153,000 links. In 2001, some Internet providers began shutting down pro-ed sites. Often this action was taken when it was determined that the sites violated the warning that the provider could do so if the sites proved to "be harmful to others." However, restriction of such Web sites is limited because of rights guaranteed by the First Amendment to the U.S. Constitution.

Congress shall make no law respecting an establishment of religion, or prohibiting the free exercise thereof; or abridging the freedom of speech, or of the press; or the right of the people peaceably to assemble, and to petition the Government for a redress of grievances.

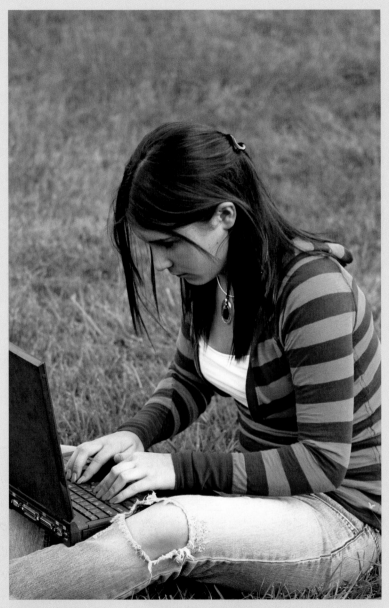

The Internet can be a valuable source of information and support when overcoming eating disorders. Unfortunately, 40% of teens visit sites that are pro-eating disorders.

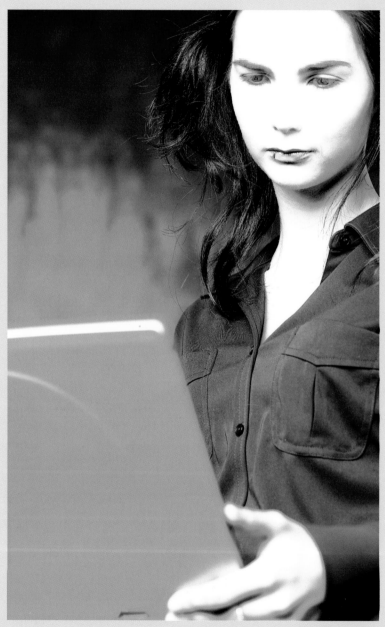

The prod-ed sites are a concern in that they might change a girl's mind about seeking treatment, or trigger a relapse.

The First Amendment to the U.S. Constitution

Few experts feel that such sites cause eating disorders, but many have expressed concern that they might discourage someone from seeking treatment or bring about a relapse. Do the administrators of pro-ana and pro-ed sites feel a sense of responsibility toward those with eating disorders? Many of the sites do open with a **disclaimer** warning viewers in treatment that it might be detrimental to their treatment for them to enter the site. Others contend they are providing a service to those with eating disorders, helping them find "healthier" ways to lose weight.

Blogs and Web sites have popped up to counteract the information provided in pro-ed sites. Visitors to those sites number far less than those who continue to visit the pro-ed sites.

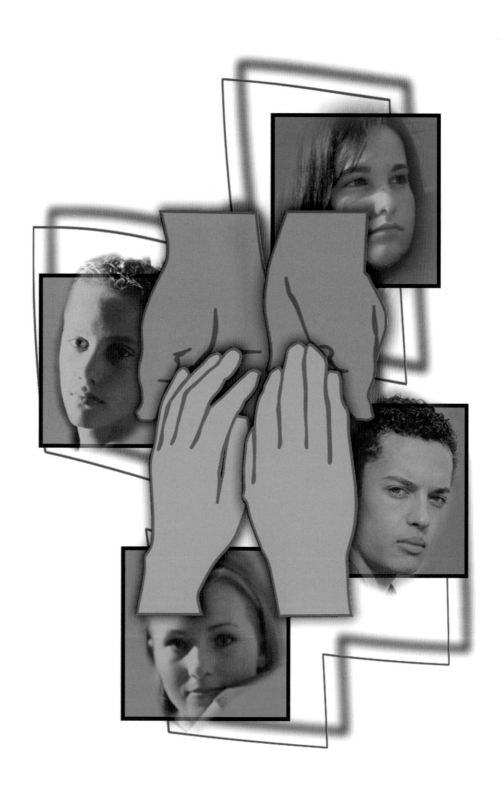

Chapter 6
Back on Track

Susan stopped at the flower shop on Grand Avenue and picked up a bouquet of flowers to take to Brooke. At first she had thought about asking Anne and Gina to go with her, but Susan decided this was something she had to do on her own. Besides, she wasn't even sure Brooke would see her.

The receptionist at the information desk gave Susan Brooke's room number and directions. Susan hesitated before opening the door. *What will she look like? Will there be tubes and machines and stuff?* Slowly, Susan opened the door and walked in. Brooke seemed to be asleep. She looked so tiny in the hospital bed. An oxygen tube threaded into her nose, and an IV tube was attached to her arm; Susan remembered those things from her father's illness. A woman sitting beside the bed turned as she heard the door open. She got up and walked toward Susan. "Hello," she said very quietly. "I'm Brooke's mom. I'm so glad you've come. Are you a friend of Brooke's?"

Not quite sure how she'd explain her relationship with Brooke, Susan just smiled and nodded. "My name is Susan. How's Brooke doing? I heard she's been pretty sick."

Brooke's mother took the flowers and put them on the table beside the bed. "Yes, she's been pretty sick, but the doctors say she'll be all right. It's just going to take a long time. I just don't understand how this happened." She sighed and slumped back in the chair, as though the weight of the entire world rested on her shoulders. "I'm afraid she's probably going to sleep through your visit. The doctor said that sleep is good for her."

"That's all right. I just wanted to stop by and see how Brooke's doing. I'll come back."

Brooke's mother took Susan's hand. "Thank you, Susan. You've been so thoughtful. I'm glad Brooke has such a good friend." Susan took a look around the room before she left. Only one other small bouquet of flowers stood on the bedside table; Susan assumed they were from Brooke's mom.

There were no balloons or cards. *I wonder if Jessica or Sydney have come by. Or Scott?*

"Susan, phone," her mother called up the stairs. Anne and Gina were in her room, so Susan didn't know who would be calling.

"Got it. Hello."

"Susan, it's Brooke." The voice was faint.

"Hi, Brooke." Gina and Anne looked up from the catalogue they'd been looking at. "How are you?"

"I'm better, Susan. Thank you for the flowers. Mom said you came by while I was asleep. I'm sorry I missed you." There was an awkward pause before she continued. "Susan, do you think you could come by this afternoon? I'd really like to talk to you."

"Sure. I'll come over around 2:30, all right?"

"You're going to go see her?" Anne asked when Susan hung up the phone. Susan nodded, expecting to hear her friends try to talk her out of it. After all, Brooke hadn't really been much of a friend to Susan. "Good," replied Anne, and Gina nodded in agreement. Susan smiled. She knew she was lucky to know true friendship.

This time when Susan opened the door to Brooke's hospital room, she was alone in the room. Smiling, Brooke motioned her to come in.

"Well, I'm glad to see you smiling," Susan told Brooke.

"I'm glad to be smiling—or doing anything else for that matter. The doctor told me I could have died."

Susan sat down in the chair hard. Though she had known that Brooke's condition was serious, hearing the words come from Brooke came as quite a shock. "How are you feeling now?"

Brooke tried to scoot up in bed, but the oxygen tube hampered her movements. "I feel better. Oh Susan, I've been so stupid." Susan reached out and touched her hand. Brooke grabbed her hand, holding it so tightly that it hurt. "I thought I was getting fat, and when you didn't have the answer—at least the one I wanted—I started doing stupid things. Laxatives, diuretics, not eating, making myself throw up, even working out for hours at a time. I could have killed myself."

Susan didn't know how to respond; she decided that sometimes it wasn't necessary to say anything.

"I even found a Web site that told me what kind of laxatives to use, how to use them, the exact—and I mean exact—calorie and fat count of almost any food available. I just didn't think I'd get so sick. And Susan," Brooke's voice dropped to a whisper, "I even tried some of the steroids that Scott uses." Brooke reached for a glass of water.

I don't know what to say to her. Should I say something? Should I just be here? What's the right thing to do?

Brooke smiled at her and gave her hand a squeeze. "I can't tell you how much it means for you to visit me. No one else has."

Susan looked around the room. The only flowers were still hers and the bouquet that had been there when she visited before. There were still no cards.

"I guess Sydney and Jessica are busy or something." Susan's heart broke to hear Brooke make excuses for her two best friends. "And Scott, well, he got into trouble when the coach found out he had steroids. If I hadn't used them, he'd have gotten away with taking them. So he's mad at me. I guess I can't blame them all."

"Brooke, don't worry about them. All you need to do is worry about getting well."

Brooke smiled. "That's the type of thing a real friend would say." This time, Susan squeezed Brooke's hand. "After I leave the hospital, I'm going to a clinic that specializes in eating disorders. I hope you can come and see me when I am allowed to have visitors."

"Try and keep me away," Susan laughed. Brooke laughed too, and the two girls were still giggling when Brooke's mother came into the room.

"I better go," Susan said. "I'll come back before you go to the 'spa.'" Brooke laughed again.

As Susan left the room, Brooke's mother whispered, "Thank you."

Susan just smiled.

As Susan walked home, she thought about how things had changed in the months since she'd returned from camp. She'd gotten off track with her weight issues, but she had taken the bull by the horns and gotten back with her plan. Susan had learned the meaning of true friendship thanks to Anne and Gina. And she'd become friends with the most popular girl in school, though not in the way she had anticipated. She laughed to herself. *Maybe we'll become the popular crowd now!*

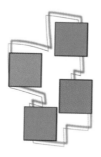

Finding Help

Admitting they have a problem is a big step for individuals with an eating disorder. The next step is to find help.

The individual should first have a physical examination to determine the extent of the problem

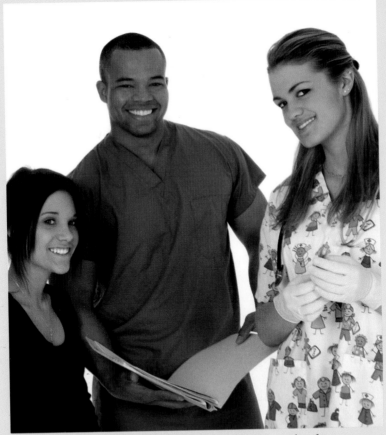

When you are ready to seek help, ask a doctor, a school nurse or a counselor for information about treatment options.

and any conditions that require immediate attention. When it's time to find a treatment program, the following can provide information and assistance in making the selection:

- doctors and nurses
- the school nurse or guidance counselor
- the local mental health agency or facility

In this cyber-age, the Internet cannot be ignored. Do a Google search for treatment methods and learn about the available options. As with any medical condition, educate yourself. Remember, though: just because something is on the Internet does not mean it is true. Use caution when researching on the Web, and stick to sites sponsored by reputable medical experts or organizations.

When It's Time to Seek Treatment

Just as with most physical and psychological conditions, treatment for an eating disorder is more successful if the condition is treated early. The longer a condition persists, the more severe will be its effects on the body and the more ingrained the disorder will be in the person's behavior.

Denial of a problem by someone with an eating disorder can make treatment difficult, even when concerned family and friends confront the individual. Someone with anorexia, for example, often does not seek treatment until an emergency situation has

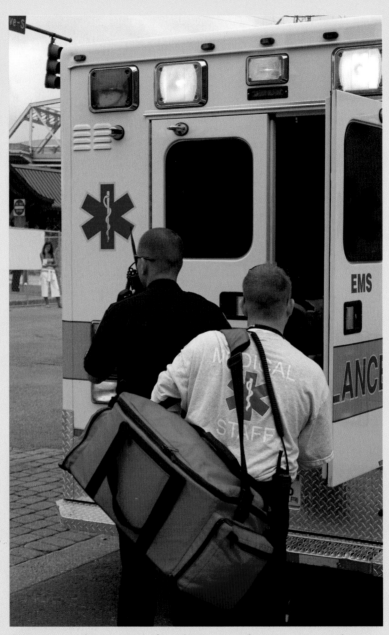

Someone with anorexia often does not seek treatment until an emergency situation brings him to the hospital.

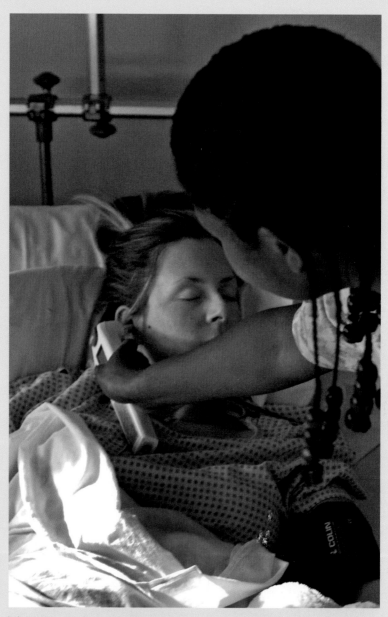

The serious physical effects of an eating disorder, such as severe weight loss or heart arrhythmias, must be dealt with before long-term treatment can begin.

brought her to the hospital. By this time, weight loss is generally severe, and the individual has had the condition for a long time. Because of the ability to hide symptoms, people with bulimia frequently have the disorder for years before seeking treatment. Individuals with binge-eating disorder often don't seek treatment until they are in their thirties and forties. Regardless of when treatment begins, it should be seen as a positive step, and people can recover from eating disorders.

Recovery begins with stabilizing the individual's condition and dealing first with the most serious problems. For the person with anorexia, for example, immediate hospitalization might be required to treat a life-threatening heart *arrhythmia* or electrolyte imbalance. Most other cases, however, can be treated on an outpatient basis.

Whatever treatment *regime* is used, the most effective recovery programs are those that combine psychiatric or psychological therapy, nutritional rehabilitation, and sometimes medication.

Drug Therapy

Over the years, drugs have been developed to aid in the treatment of psychiatric disorders. These medications have not proven to be effective in treating the eating disorder themselves. However, some have proven to be beneficial in treating coexisting conditions that occur with the eating disorder.

Anorexia and Drug Therapy

The first goal in the treatment of anorexia is to restore weight lost. Only after the physical effects of anorexia have been stabilized, can doctor, patient, family, and other members of the treatment team look for long-term methods of dealing with the disorder. Psychiatric medications have not proven to be of much help in treating anorexia.

Many individuals with anorexia are also battling depression. The connection between the two disorders is unclear; researchers have been unable to determine whether depression is the cause or effect of the eating disorder. Regardless of the connection, many with anorexia find it beneficial to take antidepressants.

Multivitamins are often prescribed to supplement nutrition, and stool softeners are used to treat constipation caused by inactive bowels.

Bulimia, Binge Eating, and Drug Therapy

The primary treatment goal for bulimia and binge-eating disorder is to reduce bingeing behaviors. Drug therapy has been more effective in treating the impulsive characteristics of bulimia and binge-eating disorder. Selective Serotonin Reuptake Inhibitors (SSRIs) such as Prozac® and Zoloft® have proven to be effective in some cases of bulimia and binge eating. This class of drugs seems to increase the amount of the neurotransmitter serotonin in the brain. This neurotransmitter has been found to be related to

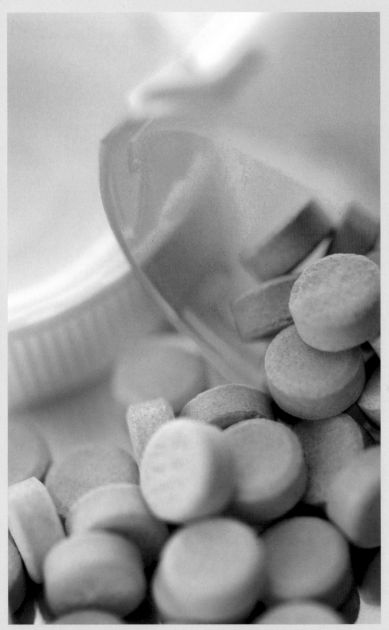

Many individuals with anorexia are also suffering from depression. These individuals benefit from taking antidepressants.

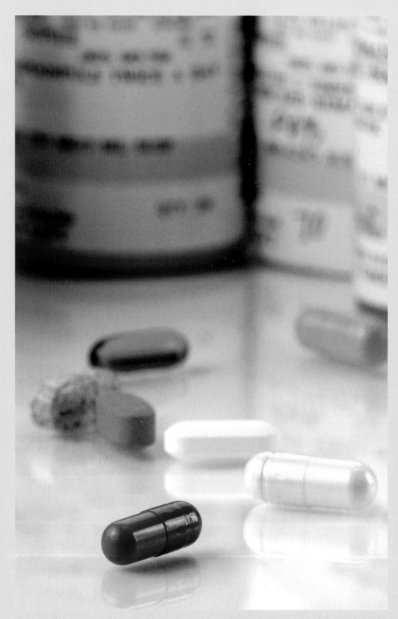

Some drugs used to treat eating disorders are not FDA approved for such usage. This "off-label" use does not mean that the drug is unsafe.

impulsivity, as well as to depression and anger, which many individuals with bulimia and binge-eating disorder experience.

Nondrug Therapy for Eating Disorders

Counseling is an important component in the treatment of eating disorders. Treating eating disorders requires unlearning behavior patterns that an individual may have practiced for many years. And as anyone who has broken a bad habit such as smoking knows, breaking habits is a hard job.

Psychodynamic psychotherapy has been effective in the treatment of anorexia. In this treatment method, individuals learn to *integrate* their feelings about their bodies, lives, and the world at large. Individuals learn ways to take control over their lives, something many attempted to find through eating disorders.

Cognitive-behavioral therapy (CBT) has proven to be an effective treatment method for eating disorders, especially bulimia and binge-eating disorder. Under CBT, people are taught the effects of their behavior. Individuals learn to change their "bad" thinking patterns and behaviors into effective ones. CBT helps people recognize their self-destructive eating habits by teaching them to gain control of their relationship with food by keeping track of their eating habits and how to change their unhealthy ones. CBT can also show individuals better ways to react to unpleasant, stressful situations, possible triggers especially for bingeing and purging episodes.

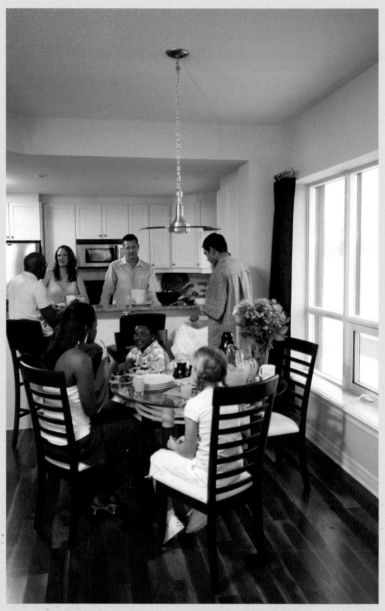

Interpersonal psychotherapy helps individuals examine and improve their relationships with family and friends.

Another therapy that has proven to be effective is interpersonal psychotherapy. This form of treatment helps individuals examine their relationships. People with eating disorders often have problems relating to family and friends. Though some of this difficulty results from the eating disorder itself, many researchers believe that relationship problems may, in some cases, lead to the development of an eating disorder.

Other Forms of Treatment

As the occurrence of eating disorders is increasing in North America, scientists are investigating other ways of treating them. Among new ways of treating eating disorders are *dialectical* behavior therapy, which helps individuals regulate emotions; the use of the antiseizure drug topiramate; exercise; and self-help techniques such as books, videos, and groups. Intensive family treatment known as the Maundsley Method is being explored also.

The Treatment Team

Helping someone overcome an eating disorder takes the expertise of many people from many areas, including the individual's family and friends. According to the American Dietetic Association (ADA; www.eatright.org), the treatment team should include:

- a doctor or advanced practice nurse familiar with eating disorders

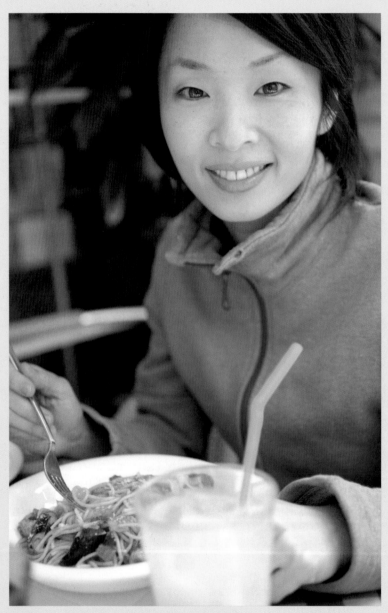

With proper treatment and the support of doctors, counselors, nutritionists, as well as family and friends, an individual can recover and lead a happy and healthy life.

- a psychotherapist or psychiatrist experienced in treating eating disorders
- a registered dietician or nutritionist with experience caring for patients with eating disorders

Eating disorders are dangerous and painful illnesses— but there is hope. With treatment, individuals who experience these disorders can once again have normal relationships with food and their bodies.

Glossary

anemia: A blood condition in which there are too few red blood cells or the red blood cells are lacking hemoglobin.

arrhythmia: An irregularity in the normal rhythm of the heart.

binge: A short period during which someone eats or drinks more than a person usually does in the same period of time.

body mass index (BMI): A measurement of body fat.

compensatory: Something done to offset the effects of something else.

criteria: Standards on which a decision is based.

dehydration: A lack of water in the body.

dialectical: Relating to the investigation of the truth through discussion.

disclaimer: A statement refusing to accept responsibility for something.

diuretics: Medications or other substances that increase the flow of urine.

electrolyte: An ion in cells, blood, or other organic material that affects most metabolic processes (such as the flow of nutrients into and waste products out of cells).

emaciated: Extremely thin, especially because of starvation or illness.

empathize: To identify with and understand another person's feelings.

esophageal: Relating to the passage down which food moves between the throat and stomach.

familial: Common to a family.

hemorrhoids: Painful varicose veins in the canal of the anus.

hypothesis: A tentative explanation for a phenomenon, used as a basis for further investigation.

impulsivity: The tendency to act on sudden urges.

integrate: To join two or more things and make a whole.

maladaptive: Unsuitable for a particular situation, function, or purpose.

metabolism: The chemical interactions in a living organism that provide the energy and nutrients necessary to sustain life.

methamphetamine: A form of highly addictive stimulant.

meticulously: Painstakingly.

musculoskeletal: Relating to the muscles and the skeleton.

neuroendocrine system: Relating to the system of cells that release a chemical messenger directly into the bloodstream.

neurotransmitters: Chemicals that carry messages between nerve cells or between nerve cells and muscles.

obsession: The uncontrollable persistence of an idea or emotion in the mind.

perfectionists: Individuals who demands perfection in all things.

prolapse: A slipping or sinking of an organ from its usual position.

purge: To rid the body of food by using laxatives or inducing vomiting.

regime: An established system of doing something.

subservience: A position of secondary importance.

Further Reading

Brinkerhoff, Shirley. *Drug Therapy and Eating Disorders.* Broomall, Pa.: Mason Crest, 2003.

Esherick, Joan. *Diet and Your Emotions: The Comfort Food Falsehood.* Broomall, Pa.: Mason Crest, 2005.

Ford, Jean. *The Truth About Diets: The Pros and Cons.* Broomall, Pa.: Mason Crest, 2005.

Gay, Kathlyn. *Am I Fat? The Obesity Issue for Teens.* Berkeley Heights, N.J.: Enslow, 2006.

Hunter, William. *How Genetics and Environment Shape Us: The Destined Body.* Broomall, Pa.: Mason Crest, 2005.

Keel, Pamela K., and Pat Levitt. *Eating Disorders.* New York: Chelsea House, 2006.

Lawton, Sandra Augustyn. *Eating Disorders Information for Teens: Health Tips About Anorexia, Bulimia, Binge Eating, and Other Eating Disorders.* Detroit, Mich.: Omnigraphics, 2005.

Libal, Autumn. *The Importance of Physical Activity and Exercise: The Fitness Factor.* Broomall, Pa.: Mason Crest, 2005.

Libal, Autumn. *Social Discrimination and Body Size: Too Big to Fit.* Broomall, Pa.: Mason Crest, 2005.

Normandi, Carol Emery, and Laurelee Roark. *Over It: A Teen's Guide to Getting Beyond Obsession with Food and Weight.* Novato, Calif.: New World Library, 2001.

Ojeda, Auriana. *Teen Decisions—Dieting.* Farmington Hills, Mich.: Greenhaven Press, 2002.

Orr, Tamra B. *When the Mirror Lies: Anorexia, Bulimia, and Other Eating Disorders.* New York: Franklin Watts, 2006.

Peacock, Judith. *Compulsive Overeating.* Mankato, Minn.: Capstone, 2000.

Shanley, Ellen, and Colleen Thompson. *Fueling the Teen Machine.* Palo Alto, Calif.: Bull Publishing, 2001.

For More Information

Body Image and Self-Esteem
www.kidshealth.org/teen/your_mind/body_image/body_
image.html

Eating Disorders
www.focusas.com/EatingDisorders.html

Eating Disorders
www.teengrowth.com

Eating Disorders: Anorexia and Bulimia
www.kidshealth.org/teen/food_fitness/problems/eat_
disorder.html

Eating for Health
www.mealsmatter.org/EatingForHealth/topics/article.
aspx?articleID=10

MEDA
www.medainc.org

National Dietetic Association
www.eatright.org

Seek Wellness
www.seekwellness.com/weight/body_image_and_you.htm

Teen Central
www.teencentral.net

Publisher's note:
The Web sites listed on this page were active at the time of publication. The publisher
is not responsible for Web sites that have changed their addresses or discontinued
operation since the date of publication. The publisher will review and update the
Web-site list upon each reprint.

Bibliography

American Psychiatric Association. *Treatment of Eating Disorders*. Arlington, Va.: 2006.

BodySense. "Eating Disorders: Not Only a Woman's Issue." http://www.bodysense.ca/parents/what_about_males_ e.html.

Consumer Health Information Service. "Eating Disorders." http://vrl.tpl.toronto.on.ca/helpfile/he_e0001.html.

Department of Health and Human Services, National Institutes of Health. "Calculate Your Body Mass Index." http://www.nhlbisupport.com/bmi.

"Facing Her Demons: High School Senior Deals with Bulimia, Issues from Her Past." *Akron (Ohio) Beacon Journal*, May 2, 2005.

Landro, Laura. "Eating Disorders on the Rise." *Chicago Sun-Times*, April 4, 2004.

National Association of Anorexia Nervosa and Associated Disorders. "Facts About Eating Disorders." http://www.anad. org/site/anadweb/content.php?type=1&id=6982.

National Center on Addiction and Substance Abuse. "Substance Abuse and Eating Disorders." http://www. casacolumbia.org.

National Institute of Mental Health. "Eating Disorders." http://www.nimh.nih.gov/publicat/eatingdisorders.cfm.

Santa Lucia, Lynn. "Driven to Be Thin." *Scholastic Choices*, September 1, 2006.

Scanlon, Bill. "Bulimia: A Threat to Body, Mind." *Rocky Mountain News (Denver, Colo.)*, August 28, 2003.

Wilson, Jenny L., Rebecka Peebles, Kristina K. Hardy, and Iris F. Litt. "Surfing for Thinness: A Pilot Study of Pro-Eating Disorder Web Site Usage in Adolescents With Eating Disorders." *Pediatrics* vol. 118(2006): 1635–1643.

Index

Picture Credits

fotolia.com
> Duplass, Jaimie: p. 107
> gdsphotography: p. 110
> Klenova, Natalie: p. 114
> Prim, Ernest: p. 109
> sonyae: p. 97

istock.com
> Allen, Darryl: p. 42
> Spanic, Damir: p. 24
> Wackerhausen, Jacob: p. 47
> Young, Lisa F.: p. 80

Jupiter Images: pp. 19, 21, 23, 26, 39, 41, 42, 48, 51, 65, 67, 68, 78, 80, 93, 94, 98, 117, 118

Author

Noa Flynn is a freelance author of many books for young adults. She lives in New York.

Series Consultants

Dr. Sara Forman graduated from Barnard College and Harvard Medical School. She completed her residency in pediatrics at Children's Hospital of Philadelphia and a fellowship in adolescent medicine at Children's Hospital, Boston (CHB). She currently is an attending physician in adolescent medicine at CHB, where she has served as director of the Adolescent Outpatient Eating Disorders Program for the past 12 years. She has also consulted for the National Eating Disorder Screening Project on their high school initiative and has presented at many conferences about teens and eating disorders. In addition to her clinical and administrative roles in the Eating Disorders Program, Dr. Forman teaches medical students and residents and coordinates the Adolescent Medicine rotation at CHB. Dr. Forman sees primary care adolescent patients in the Adolescent Clinic at CHB, at Bentley College, and at the Germaine Lawrence School, a residential school for emotionally disturbed teenage girls.

Cindy Croft, M.A.Ed., is the Director of the Center for Inclusive Child Care (CICC) at Concordia University, St. Paul, MN. The CICC is a comprehensive resource network for promoting and supporting inclusive early childhood and school-age programs and providers with Project EXCEPTIONAL training and consultation, and other resources at www.inclusivechildcare. org. In addition to working with the CICC, Ms. Croft is on the faculty at Concordia University and Minneapolis Community and Technical College.